HEALTHY HIPS HANDBOOK

EXERCISES FOR TREATING AND PREVENTING COMMON HIP JOINT INJURIES

DR. KARL KNOPF

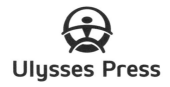

Ulysses Press

Published in the United States by
Ulysses Press
P.O. Box 3440
Berkeley, CA 94703
www.ulyssespress.com

ISBN: 978-1-56975-819-9
Library of Congress Control Number 2010925859

Printed in Canada by Webcom

10 9 8 7 6 5 4 3 2 1

Acquisitions: Keith Riegert
Managing editor: Claire Chun
Editor: Lily Chou
Proofreader: Lauren Harrison
Production: Judith Metzener, Abigail Reser
Cover design: what!design @ whatweb.com
Cover photographs: © Rapt Productions
Interior photographs: © Rapt Productions except page 11 © Linda Bucklin/
    shutterstock.com and page 12 © YorkBerlin/shutterstock.com
Models: Brian Goodell, Toni Silver and Karl Knopf

Distributed by Publishers Group West

Please Note
This book has been written and published strictly for informational purposes, and in no way should be used as a substitute for actual instruction with qualified professionals. The author and publisher are providing you with information in this work so that you can have the knowledge and can choose, at your own risk, to act on that knowledge. The author and publisher also urge all readers to be aware of their health status and to consult health care professionals before beginning any health program.

table of contents

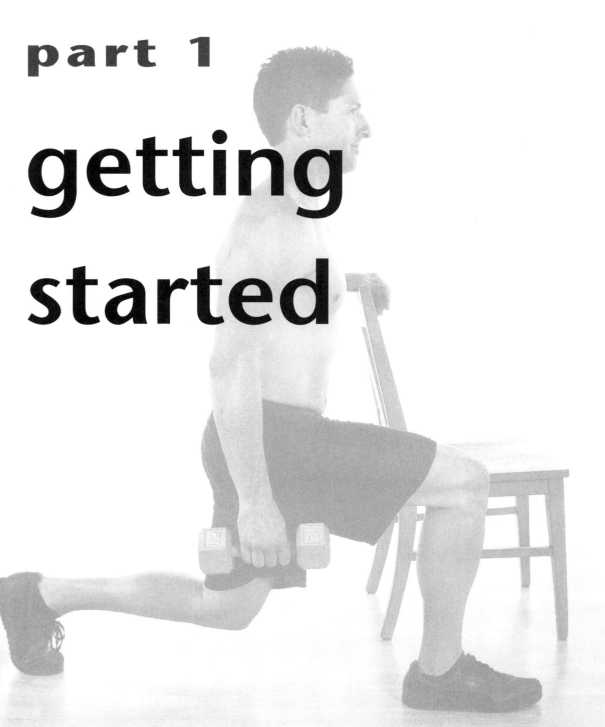

part 1
getting
started

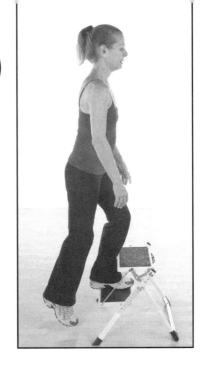

introduction

The hip plays an important role in many everyday activities, from sitting down to climbing stairs to bending over and touching your toes. The hip joint withstands forces about one-third of your body weight while you're standing, three times your body weight when you walk up stairs, and increases significantly to four times your body weight when you run. This means anyone, regardless of age or fitness level, may experience a hip problem at some point in their lives.

The pelvis supports the spine and trunk and transfers their weight to the lower limbs. The pelvis is the anchor for many torso muscles as well as leg muscles. The hip joint is formed where the neck of the femur (upper leg bone) connects with the pelvis; the hip is a deep ball-and-socket joint that is very stable and capable of carrying heavy loads. When we look at the anatomy of the hip region, we'll see the interconnectedness of the pelvic region, low back and upper leg. Bones intersect, muscles cross over each joint area, and nerve roots are very close to each other.

The thigh, hip and pelvis area generally have less incidence of injuries than do the knee and ankle. Yet, the hip and pelvic area do suffer a great deal of trauma, bruises and chronic misuse, not to mention even occasional abuse. Unfortunately, most people don't feel the effects of the misuse and abuse until it's too late.

When we discuss hip problems, we're referring to the tendons, ligaments, bursa, joint articulations and muscles of the hip area. *Healthy Hips Handbook* is designed to help prevent a hip problem for some and, for those of you with existing hip problems, provide post-rehabilitation exercises that you and your health-care provider can select to best meet your needs. The focus of this book is to encourage you to take time to rethink your motions and to better understand that the structure under your skin is not invincible. What you do today has a significant bearing on how you'll feel tomorrow. As one former professional athlete said late in life, when he was limping around, "If I knew I was going to live this long, I would've taken better care of myself!" When we're young, we think nothing will ever happen to us, and if it does some doctor will just fix it. While medical science is wonderful, nothing is ever as good as the original. Please do whatever is necessary today to maintain your body's warranty.

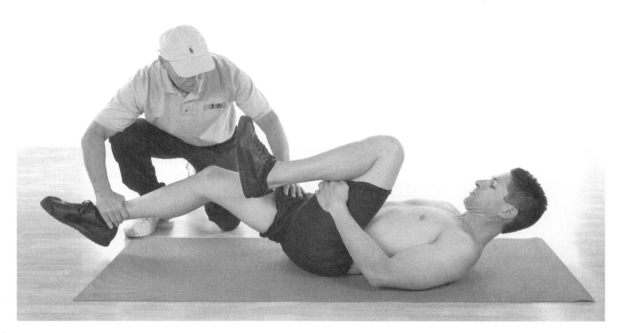

Author Karl Knopf makes some adjustments.

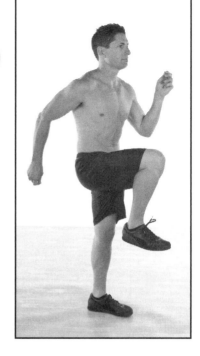

anatomy of the hip joint

Understanding how the hip functions will provide insight into how to better care for it. Often called the workhorse of the joints, the hip is a ball-and-socket joint: the head of the upper leg is the ball and where it connects inside the pelvis is the socket.

This design allows for a very diverse set of actions, including flexion (bringing your knee to your chest), extension (swinging your leg behind you), adduction (bringing your legs together), abduction (raising your leg to the side), circumduction (circling your leg) and rotation. These actions are vital in the activities of daily living, ambulation, and recreation and sports.

Bones and Joints

Although the hip joint is similar to the shoulder joint in design, the hip joint is structurally more stable and better protected. The neck of the upper leg bone (the femur) rests deep inside the pelvis, whereas the shoulder joint is like a golf tee lying on its side next to a golf ball, with its structure held in place by bands called tendons and ligaments.

The large, flat, irregular-shaped pelvis is the supporting structure of the hip joint and made up of a ring of three bones: the *ilium*, *ischium* and *pubis*. At the base of the spine are the *sacrum* and the *coccyx*; as the human ages, these two fuse with the rear of the pelvis. The pelvis provides a solid insert for the leg to connect to the upper body, to support the spine and to transfer the load to the legs. This solid base serves as the origin and insertion point for many muscles. The female pelvis is wider than the male pelvis and designed for child bearing, so the shape of a woman's hip is different from a man's.

The actual joint is where the "ball" of the upper leg, or *femur*, fits into the *acetabulum*, or socket, deep within the pelvis. This is what provides the hip joint with the most support. The rim of the joint is surrounded by a protective sheath called the *glenoid labrum*, or fibrocartilage; cartilage covers the head of the femur. The capsule is lined with *synovial membrane* and several ligaments. The synovial membrane provides lubrication, as do several fluid-filled sacs called *bursas*. The ligaments provide additional support. The *iliofemoral ligament* is the strongest attachment in the human body. Its primary functions are to prevent hyperextension of the hip, limit external rotation of the hip and limit adduction of the femur. The iliofemoral ligament also limits adduction of the femur as well as excessive internal rotation of

the hip. The *pubofemoral ligament* prevents excessive abduction of the femur. The joint's design, with its bone structure, ligaments and muscular attachments, makes the hip the powerhouse joint of the body.

Muscles

Muscles around the hip joint help take some of the load off the joint structure itself. In addition, they support your body weight and absorb the shock of movement.

The gluteal region is composed of the buttocks and hip area. Several muscles make up this region. The *gluteus maximus*, as the name implies, is the biggest part of your rear end. This powerful muscle extends the upper leg and laterally rotates the thigh. If you place your hand on your rear end and perform a squat, you'll feel your gluteus maximus engaging. The *gluteus medius* is a medium-sized muscle in your rear end; it's used for abduction and internal rotation

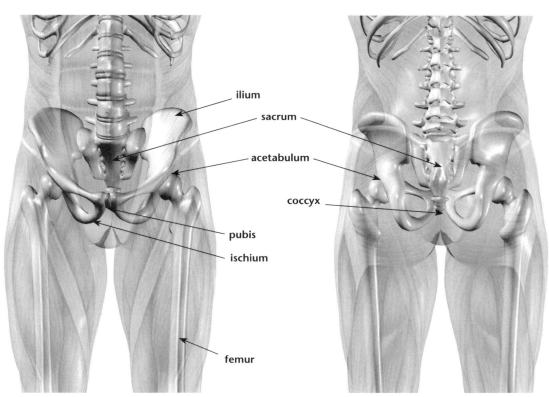

ilium
sacrum
acetabulum
coccyx
pubis
ischium
femur

Major bones of the hips

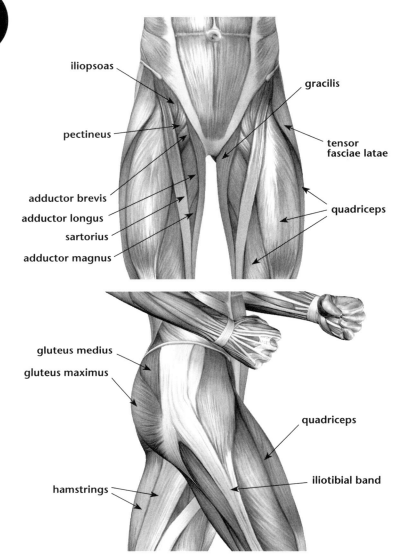

iliopsoas

gracilis

pectineus

tensor
fasciae latae

adductor brevis

adductor longus

quadriceps

sartorius

adductor magnus

gluteus medius

gluteus maximus

quadriceps

iliotibial band

hamstrings

Major muscles that affect the hips; note that some muscles (such as the obturators and piriformis) lie beneath large surface muscles such as the gluteus maximus

Obturator internus—This muscle is responsible for rotating the thigh outward.

Pectineus—This muscle acts as a flexor and an adductor of the leg.

Psoas major and minor—Along with the *iliacus*, these two powerful muscles share a common insertion and act synergistically. Commonly called the iliopsoas muscle, they work in concert to flex the thigh and flex the torso at the hip joint.

Adductor longus, brevis and magnus—These three muscles all work to adduct the leg.

Tensor fasciae latae—This muscle assists with flexion and internal rotation of the upper leg.

The pelvis serves as the anchor for many muscles, such as the *quadriceps* at the front of the thigh and the *hamstrings* at the rear of the leg, which assist in leg motion. Without a solid platform to attach to, the quads and hamstrings would not be able to function.

of the thigh. A yet smaller portion of the rear end, the *gluteus minimus* internally rotates the thigh and helps in abducting the thigh.

Other muscles play a role in the hip joint:

Piriformis—This small, intrinsic muscle lies deep within the hip area. It externally rotates the thigh and assists in extending and abducting it.

Obturator externus—This muscle rotates the thigh externally.

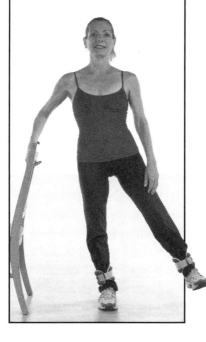

common hip issues

Many people, from the very active to the very old, suffer from hip problems. All too often a person with a hip problem also has a back issue. Experts believe that seven major factors play a role in hip problems: muscle imbalances of the hip, low back and upper leg; asymmetrical issues of gait and leg length; poor posture; improper muscle recruitment; trauma or injury; misuse and abuse (wear and tear); and nerve impingement.

When the muscles supporting the hip region become weak, more of the load has to be transmitted to the already compromised joint, which in turn increases pain, thus creating a vicious circle. Most people in pain don't want to exercise, but strong muscles can be a key factor in both improving function as well as decreasing pain. Keep in mind, however, that chronic misuse of the joint will at some point manifest as an injury, especially if you're biomechanically predisposed to injury.

Some hip issues are brought on by overuse; basically, people dismiss little irritations and continue to train through them, leading to major issues later. Overuse syndromes often result when a person changes his routine, whether by playing more sets of tennis, running longer distances or trying a different dance routine.

Prevention is the best treatment, so early intervention on a small problem is always the prudent thing to do. This is why having a hip issue diagnosed early by a health professional is highly suggested. If a small problem is not addressed at the onset of pain or discomfort, it can become a chronic issue. While the Internet is a wonderful tool to gather information, too many people use it to self-diagnose themselves. This book recommends that you always get a medical evaluation before you try to treat yourself. After a consultation with a medical professional, you can better understand your course of action.

The following is by no means a comprehensive list of hip concerns, nor is the intent of this section to provide you with a means of self-evaluation. Always consult your primary care physician to determine what your specific issue is, and remember that the hip region can manifest pain from numerous sources other than the hip itself.

General Anatomic Impairments

The design of the hip has a significant influence on how it tolerates wear and tear. There are two basic anatomic design flaws that influence how your hip will perform:

- Angle of inclination and torsion, which is basically the angle at which the neck of the femur connects to the pelvic area.
- Leg length discrepancy, which is often the result of functional relationships of the spine, the pelvis and the long bones of the leg, as well as the foot. Leg length discrepancy can result in hip and knee pain.

While these two issues might not be visible to the eye, habitual use of a slightly off-center alignment can cause major problems over time, such as muscle strains and tendonitis, as well as groin strain.

Muscle strains and tears can also occur when people stretch a "cold" muscle without being warmed up, perform bouncing or "ballistic" stretches, overstretch beyond their normal limits or perform explosive activities such as sprinting.

There are three categories of tears:

Grade 1 strain—This category involves the least amount of pain and discomfort. Often, the thigh just feels "tight."

Grade 2 strain—At this level, the person feels a "pulling sensation" and recognizes that something is not right, but often neglects the signs and still trains. The problem can then escalate into a grade 3 strain.

Grade 3 strain—This is serious because the muscle really pulls apart or ruptures. If the person feels a "pop," it's time to see a medical doctor.

Groin Strain

Groin strains are very common and seen often in female runners due to the anatomical differences between men and women. A woman's wider pelvis causes her foot to turn inward (pronate) when running, which sets her up for pulled muscles. Groin strains first appear as minor issues; however, if not addressed early they can become chronic issues that can take an inordinate amount of time to heal. They are often difficult to treat and can easily be aggravated even after the person feels they are healed.

The groin includes the following muscles: gracilis, pectineus and adductor group (brevis, longus and/or magnus). These muscles are relatively small players in the hip area and are often neglected in conditioning programs. Often the best treatment for a groin strain is just resting the area and using alternative means to stay fit. Your doctor may suggest swimming, arm-crank bikes or water walking.

Symptoms

- Sudden twinge in the upper inside portion of the leg
- Pain and/or weakness in the upper inside portion of the leg
- Internal bleeding, in severe cases

Common Causes

- Explosive movements such as running or jumping
- Muscle imbalances
- External rotation of the leg, such as weaving through a line of cones

Treatment

- RICE (rest, ice, compression, elevation)
- Whirlpool treatment
- Cryotherapy (ice massage)
- Ultrasound
- Corrective exercises (strength and flexibility)
- Wrapping
- Biomechanics evaluation
- Active rest
- Water therapy
- Watchful waiting

Bursitis

The specific term for this condition is *trochanteric bursitis*. The source of pain is a little fluid-filled sac called the bursa. The sac acts as a cushion between the bones and the tendons. Basically, bursitis is the inflammation of the bursa sac.

Symptoms

- Pain or discomfort, typically on the outside area of the hip
- Pain made worse when lying on your side, climbing stairs, or sitting or standing for too long

Common Causes

- Overuse of the hip joint (overtraining)
- Misuse of the hip joint and doing movements that are biomechanically incorrect.
- Abuse of the hip joint by doing activities that are extremely challenging to the hip area and cause an injury
- Females who have a pronounced "Q" angle (the angle from the outside of the pelvic bone to the midpoint on the knee) are at greater risk

- Leg length discrepancies
- Arthritis
- Abnormal gait
- Muscle imbalances

Treatment

- Rest
- Abstinence from activities that cause pain, such as running, standing and bending
- Leg length evaluation
- "Q" angle evaluation
- RICE (rest, ice, compression, elevation)
- Corrective exercises (stretching and strengthening)
- Anti-inflammatory medications
- Ice and/or heat packs

Snapping Hip

Snapping hip is very much like the name implies. This condition is often seen in dancers,

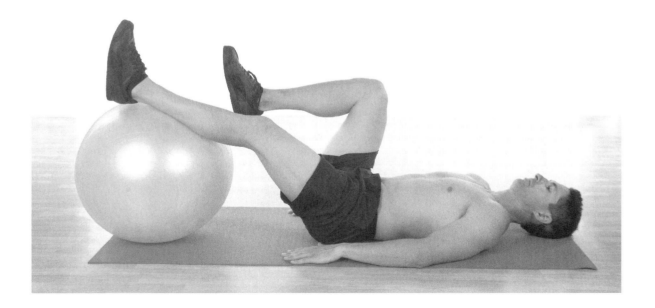

gymnasts, hurdlers or people who perform pronounced hip and leg movements, where the leg is taken to extreme ranges of motions quickly and ballistically.

Symptoms

- A snapping sensation or sound in or around the hip joint
- Pain in the hip region
- Snapping in the hip joint when standing on one leg

Common Causes

- Bad body mechanics
- Muscle imbalances
- Hip instability

Treatment

- RICE (rest, ice, compression, elevation)
- Active rest
- Eliminating contributing factors and activities

- Biomechanical assessment
- Medical intervention
- Corrective exercise, like stretching and conditioning exercises or hydrotherapy

Iliotibial Band Fasciitis

The ITB or IT band is a belt of fibrous tissues that runs on the outside of the upper leg from the hip to the knee. ITB syndrome is an overuse syndrome due to repeated friction (flexion) of the ITB against the outside of the bony protrusion (epicondyle) of the femur, which irritates the underlying bursa. Sometimes ITB syndrome is mistaken for sciatica, and some people may have associated trochanteric bursitis.

Symptoms

- Pain along the outside of the thigh

- Pain over the buttocks
- Pain down the back of the leg and below the knee

Common Causes

- Inflammation of the ITB
- Trochanter bursitis causing pressure on the ITB
- Faulty biomechanics
- Muscle imbalances
- Overuse

Treatment

- Abstinence from activities that cause discomfort, like running or cycling
- Deep-tissue massage
- Anti-inflammatory medications
- Cryotherapy (ice massage)
- Electric stimulation/ ultrasound
- Corrective stretches
- Muscle re-patterning

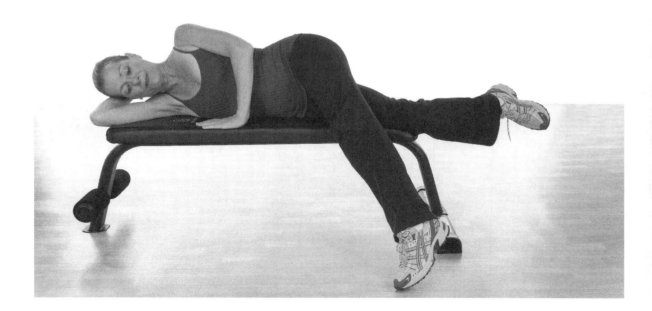

- Taping
- Ambulation aides, such as canes

Sciatic Pain

The sciatic nerve is the longest and widest nerve in the human body. Sciatic pain is caused by compression or irritation of the sciatic nerve. Some experts believe that if the sciatic nerve gets pinched where it runs through the piriformis muscle, it can replicate the sciatic pain caused by a herniated disc of the lower back. A common sign is if the pain is made worse when you sit on your wallet. In this case, it may be caused by a tight piriformis muscle.

Symptoms
- Pain down your leg and near your buttock

Common Causes
- Tight piriformis muscle
- Herniated disc

Treatment
- Stretching routine that targets the piriformis muscle
- Health consultation to rule out a herniated disc

Traumatic Conditions

Hip Dislocation

Hip dislocations, the result of major trauma to the pelvic region, are fairly rare, but they're serious medical conditions that require immediate medical attention. Following the acute medical intervention treatment, a comprehensive physical therapy treatment plan should be implemented.

Symptoms
- Dislocation is visible or palpable

Common Causes
- Forceful impact

Treatment
- Immediate hospitalization in case of shock and internal damage

Hip Pointers

Hip pointers are seen in people who are involved in sports such as soccer and football, where collisions and impacts occur to the rim of the pelvis, which cause bruising to bone and associated soft tissue. The area that is impacted usually has a bad-looking bruise and is sore to the touch.

Symptoms
- Immediate and severe pain on the tip of the hip bone, by the belt line (iliac crest)

Common Causes
- Trauma to the iliac crest

Treatment
- Treatment of pain and spasms
- RICE (rest, ice, compression, elevation)
- Ultrasound
- Protective padding

Osteitis Pubis

Osteitis pubis is found in people who are involved in sports with a large amount of lower-body movement, such as distance running, soccer, football, rugby and martial arts. Repetitive motions can cause an inflammatory response in the muscles and soft tissue in that area.

Symptoms
- Tenderness in the pelvic region where impact occurred (often the top of the hip bone)
- Pain when performing sit-ups, running or squatting motions

Common Causes
- Overuse
- Misuse

Treatment
- RICE (rest, ice, compression, elevation)
- Rest
- Medications and ultrasound
- Alternative training routines
- Correction of poor body mechanics
- Correction of muscle imbalances

Degenerative Joint Disease (DJD)

Also called arthritis or osteoarthritis, this condition of the hip can wreak havoc on your quality of life. Osteoarthritis is the most common form of arthritis in the United States. Arthritis of the hip occurs in 3 percent of people older than 30 years of age. It increases with age, often affecting more women than men. The causes of arthritis are multifactoral and include biomechanical

as well as biochemical issues. Genetics, diet, estrogen and bone density, along with joint looseness, obesity and lack of muscle, are all contributors. However, age is not a cause of osteoarthritis. While osteoarthritis is more commonly seen in older adults, much joint discomfort is the result of *how* we've lived rather than *how long*. The severity of DJD ranges from mild to severe. In severe cases, joint replacement may be an option. As with all of these conditions, diagnosis of DJD should be made by a physician.

Symptoms
- Inflammation
- Joint stiffness
- Pain
- "Grinding" in the hip area

Possible Causes
- Wear and tear (misuse and abuse)
- Misaligned joints
- Excessive body weight
- Poor body mechanics
- Previous injury

Treatment
- Lifestyle modification (stay fit, lean and healthy)
- Corrective exercises (stretching and strengthening)
- Anti-inflammatory medication
- Steroid injections
- Water exercise

- Active rest
- Gentle range of motion
- Ice or heat applications
- Ambulation aids such as canes, walkers or wheelchairs
- Surgery
- Patient education

Pelvic Girdle Fractures

As noted in the anatomy section on page 10, the pelvis is the bony ring formed by the sacrum and the coccyx; it's designed to support the upper body. The hip is where the neck of the femur (long bone of the upper leg) connects to the pelvis via the ball-and-socket joint. Pelvic fractures are rare and are caused by severe trauma, such as a car accident or fall. A fracture of the neck of the femur (commonly referred to as a broken hip), however, is more common. For older people, this is one of the most feared injuries, and for good reason—it can contribute to disability and death. One in two women over 50 years of age and one in eight men over 50 has osteoporosis. One in five people over 50 years of age who breaks a hip dies within one year because the prolonged bed rest after the injury leads to many health problems. A stress fracture at the hip is more subtle than a pelvic girdle fracture. Stress fractures are often called "hair-line" cracks in the thigh bone and are often caused by overtraining. Sometimes stress fractures are undiagnosed or misdiagnosed as muscle strain or tendonitis.

If you suspect someone has a pelvic bone fracture or broken femur, consult emergency personnel immediately. The person is at risk for going into shock as a result of internal bleeding. Do not move the person, if possible; placing the person in a weight-bearing stance can cause additional damage.

Symptoms
- Severe pain in the pelvis/hip area
- Inability to stand

Common Causes
- Blunt force trauma
- Severe impact trauma
- Osteoporosis
- Frailty (poor reactions, lack of muscle strength)

Treatment
Treatment is often bed rest, which can contribute to a whole host of medical problems. Unfortunately, surgery is not possible due to the fact that the fracture of the neck of the femur is like putting a puzzle back together and the structure of the neck of the femur is often affected by osteoporosis. A physical therapist will establish a home-based treatment plan that

focuses on preventing further functional loss and blood clots. An occupational therapist will evaluate assistant devices needed for activities of daily living.

Hip Conditions Seen in Children

Although this book focuses on adult conditions, many so-called minor injuries, if not addressed early on and corrected, can manifest themselves as painful chronic conditions later in life. Therefore, if you're responsible for the well-being of children, you may want to be aware of the following conditions.

Legg Calve Perthe Disease (LCPD)

LCPD is a flattening of the femoral head (top of the leg bone), which limits the range of motion of the hip in the socket. This avascular necrosis of the femoral head generally occurs in children between 3 and 12 years of age, and more often in active boys.

Symptoms
- Pain along the inside of the leg and into the knee area

Common Causes
- Unknown

Treatment
- Corrective stretching and strengthening exercises
- Bracing
- Surgery

Slipped Capital Femoral Epiphysis

This condition, in which the ball of the hip joint slips from the femur, is most often found in boys aged 10 to 17 who are generally very tall and thin or obese. While the cause of the condition is unknown, often it's related to the effects of growth hormone.

Symptoms
- Only minimal pain early on; more pronounced pain in hip and knee during most motions (passive and active) as stages advance
- Limited range of motion in abduction, flexion and internal rotation
- Pain in the groin as a result of trauma
- Outward-turned leg

Common Causes
- Unknown, but possibly related to growth hormone released during a growth spurt, as well as trauma and falls.

Treatment
- Reduced weight bearing
- In severe cases, surgery

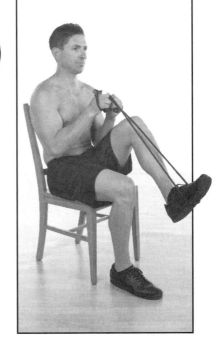

hip rehab

The hip joint is very complex and often pain in that area can be referred from another unrelated part of the body, such as the lower back, or even from an infection. The hip joint has its own blood and nerve supply, and it's not uncommon for hip pain to be referred from the spinal area. This is why a complete health history and medical work-up should be done by a physician. Self-diagnosis is not a wise idea.

Generally, pain and/or loss of function is the first sign that something is going on. Unless you suffer a traumatic injury such as a dislocation, usually the first step of your treatment will be visiting your primary care physician, who may refer you to an orthopedic or neurological specialist. The doctor will most likely sit down with you and discuss the signs and symptoms of your condition.

Additionally, the doctor will take a case history (to find out when it hurts, what makes it feel worse or better, and what might have caused the problem), observe your gait, observe your range of motion and palpate the affected areas.

Some doctors may have you perform some functional movements as well and muscle-test you. If the doctor feels you warrant further evaluation, he may refer you for more tests, such as an MRI or another type of radiological exam, to rule out any serious health issues. Some doctors may even look for leg length discrepancies or postural deviations.

When you're speaking with your doctor, be as specific as possible when describing your pain (is it sharp and stabbing, is it just a dull ache, does it feel like there's snapping or grinding?). The three general classifications of injury are:

MILD—At this stage, the doctor may recommend a home-based exercise program that includes corrective exercise and specific stretches. Keep in mind that you're still injured and re-injury is very common. Do not rush the body's healing.

MODERATE—At this stage, passive and light active range-of-motion exercises may be advised. Protective rest of the joint, as well as modalities to control pain, will be recommended.

SEVERE—At this stage, rest, ice and heat applications, and

range-of-motion exercises are often recommended. Pain management options such as medications or possible injections can be discussed. Preventing further damage is critical. Attempting to "play through" pain and dismissing your injury will only prolong the rehabilitation process. Avoid movements such as bringing your knee into your chest past 90 degrees and swinging your leg too far out to the side. Restoration of hip function should address both the local and general effects of the injury and comprehensively treat both the injury and the whole body.

Note that the absence of symptoms does not mean full restoration. Just treating the injury and neglecting the total person will set the individual up for another injury. In athletes, 30 to 50 percent of all sports injuries are related to overuse or improper training techniques. Some studies have shown that 27 percent of these injuries are re-injuries, and that 16 percent occurred within one month of returning to play. Also, remember the two-hour rule: If you hurt more than two hours after an exercise session, you need to reduce activity to a level that does not cause pain; if you continue to hurt or lose range of motion,

consult your doctor ASAP. An effective rehabilitation routine will train both the brain and the body, which is why you need to be mindful when training. In today's managed health care, physical therapists often don't have time to fully attend to all the aspects needed for complete restoration. This is why you play a significant part in restoring yourself to full function.

The Therapy Process

After a complete work-up, the doctor will devise a treatment plan for your condition. Some of the options include watchful waiting, rest and meditation, physical therapy, injections or, in severe cases, surgical intervention. If you follow the program exactly, it will hasten your return to full function.

The rehabilitation goals occur in three stages: acute, recovery and function.

Phase 1: Acute Stage

The acute stage focuses on preventing further harm, decreasing the signs and symptoms of injury, and hastening the healing process. A trained therapist should oversee this phase of rehabilitation. Take this book along with you to your medical appointment and have your

---

TYPES OF INJURIES

Knowing the cause of an injury is critical in developing a comprehensive rehabilitation program. Some injuries are the result of a sudden impact; others are the result of chronic misuse, overuse or abuse of the body or body parts. Generally speaking, there are two types of injury, macro trauma and micro trauma.

Macro trauma is an injury due to a specific event. The time, place and mechanism of injury are usually quite clear. The single event results in a previously normal/healthy structure becoming suddenly and distinctly abnormal after the event (e.g., hip separation).

Micro traumas are chronic, repetitive injuries. These injuries actually arise from misalignments and poor body mechanics combined with repetitive insults to the area. Chronic conditions, unlike acute injuries, must be managed and cannot be quickly resolved.

---

health care provider choose specific exercises from our selection.

The goals of Phase 1 are to:
- Manage pain
- Maintain range of motion
- Maintain neuromuscular control
- Prevent muscle atrophy and functional loss.

The criteria for advancement to Phase 2 are:
- Controlled pain
- Evidence of healing

- Near-normal range of motion
- Exercise tolerance

Phase 2: Recovery Phase

This phase can be done with an adaptive-fitness personal trainer or by yourself—as long as you or your trainer stays within the scope of practice and follows the protocols set forth by the medical professional. At this stage, many people re-injure themselves by pushing themselves too hard and not heeding their bodies. So be careful and patient.

The goals of Phase 2 are to:

- Prevent further injury and pain
- Regain lower body strength, muscular balance and pelvic stability
- Foster hip flexibility
- Improve neuromuscular control and coordination

The criteria for advancement to Phase 3 are:

- No pain, especially no additional pain from exercise intervention
- Complete tissue healing
- Almost complete range of motion
- Near-normal strength when compared to the uninvolved side (approximately 75 to 80 percent)

Phase 3: Function Phase

This phase can be done with an adaptive fitness personal trainer or by yourself—as long as you or your trainer stays within the scope of practice and follows the protocols set forth by the medical professional. Once you've regained full functional recovery, evaluate the circumstances that may have caused your condition and adapt your lifestyle and behaviors. By being sensible, following your therapist's suggestions and participating in the exercises included in this book, you reduce your chances of re-injuring yourself.

The goals of Phase 3 are to:

- Learn the importance of proper training techniques and body mechanics in daily activities
- Learn how to exercise the stabilizing muscles of the pelvic area and learn proper posture and lifestyle changes to prevent future injury
- Increase muscular strength and endurance in preparation for work or sports demands
- Improve multi-plane range of motion
- Institute sport-specific drills and functional weight-transfer and weight-bearing activities of daily living (i.e., weight shifts)
- Be evaluated to see if you're ready to re-engage in a fully active lifestyle

The criteria for knowing you've reached "full functional recovery" are:

- Zero pain
- Full and completely pain-free engagement in activities

self-massage series

Massage is the process of manipulating the body's soft tissues using methods such as friction, vibration and stroking. The goal of massage is to relax the muscle or in some cases invigorate it. Often, a massage increases blood flow to that area. By placing sustained pressure on the area, the adhesion will lengthen and release the tension. Performing self-massage can prepare the joint for motion or provide relief after an exercise/therapy session. It decreases soft tissue adhesions, increasing range of motion and flexibility. It also decreases muscle soreness. Self-massage is best performed when the muscle is warm. Here we use the foam roller (available at various local retailers, including medical suppliers, yoga/Pilates studios and sporting goods stores) and the standard tennis ball. Acute and chronic pain can be caused by "trigger points." A trigger point is a specific sensitive area that's painful. They may have a small surface area but are hyperirritable. When performing a self-massage, try to locate the trigger point, which will be easy to find because it's often painful to the touch. Press on the area for 5–30 seconds or as long as is tolerated.

foam roller   *quads*

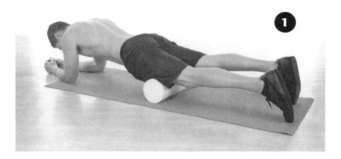

1 Lie face down with the fronts of your thighs on the roller.

2 Roll back and forth between your hips and your knees, but do not roll over your knees. If you find an especially tight spot, stop for a moment and breathe until the muscle softens and the tightness/discomfort diminishes.

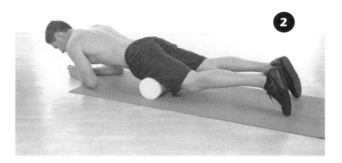

foam roller

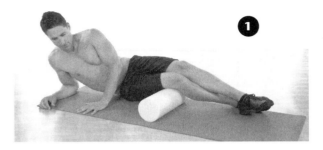

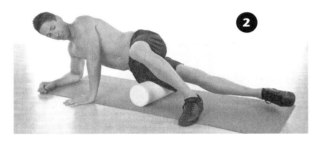

1 Lie on your side, propping yourself up on one arm and placing the roller on the outside of your bottom leg.

2 Roll back and forth between your hips and your knees, but do not roll over your knees. If you find an especially tight spot, stop for a moment and breathe until the muscle softens and the tightness/discomfort diminishes. For additional balance, you can place your top foot on the floor in front of you.

foam roller

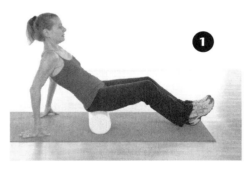

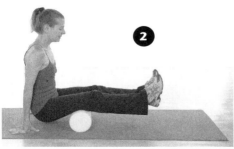

1 Sit on the roller with your hands on the floor behind you.

2 Roll back and forth between your bottom and your knees, breathing comfortably, allowing the tightness/discomfort to release. If you lack upper body strength, you can perform this one leg at a time.

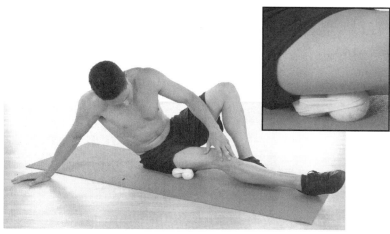

1 Place the tennis ball(s) under the point of discomfort. Roll back and forth to release tension.

IT band

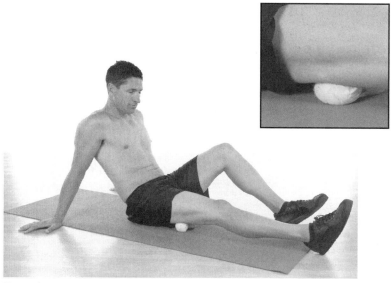

Hamstrings

part 2
prevention
& programs

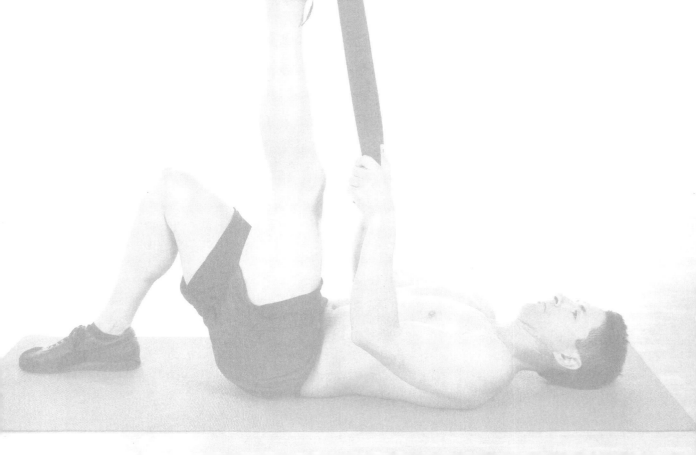

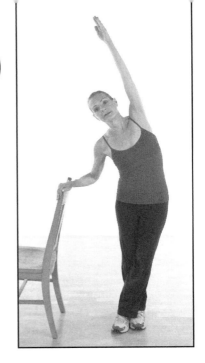

preventing re(injury)

Rehabilitation of the hip is a difficult, painful process, and sometimes the person never fully recovers. A former chief of orthopedic surgery once told me that surgeons can do remarkable things and the hardware for hip replacements is much better today than ever before, but it's never as good as the original equipment. Therefore, the message is prevention: It's always cheaper to prevent an injury than to treat it.

The best defense against a hip problem is to stay proactive. This involves a comprehensive strengthening and stretching program for the total hip region. It's never too late to get better.

Muscle imbalances are incredibly common in the fitness and athletic arenas—the more we exercise, the greater those imbalances become. We're designed with muscles that opposed each other to create a symmetrical body. Unfortunately, as a result of our lifestyle (e.g., most of the sports we participate in, such as golf, racquetball and softball, are done in an asymmetrical or one-sided manner), we've disturbed this delicate balance. Inflexible muscles often get tighter and weak muscles become even weaker, increasing the potential for injury. Any time you sit, stand, jump, run, bike or swim, your hip joint is activated. Chronic misuse of the joint will at some point manifest as an injury, especially if you're biomechanically predisposed to injury. Therefore, to recover from or to prevent an injury we need to create a more balanced body.

All the physical therapy in the world won't help if you continue to habitually engage in poor body mechanics. Each muscle has been designed with a specific role in mind. Some are prime actors while others play supporting roles, and they often fluctuate between major player and helper. We get into trouble when we ask a muscle to do a job that another is better designed to perform. When this occurs, we see muscles rebel by going into spasm and shutting down. It's extremely difficult to re-pattern your muscles and re-teach them to "fire" only when they're supposed to and to relax when a more appropriate muscle should be taking the lead role. Having an ergonomics expert evaluate your standing and sitting postures as well as your gait is a good idea.

Consider the following tips for healthier hips:

1. A moderate dose of corrective exercise will keep muscles from becoming weak and placing undue load on the other joints of the body's kinetic chain.
2. A gentle dose of regular exercise keeps the joints lubricated.
3. Regular exercise is a necessity for anyone desiring optimal functional performance in sports or activities of daily living.

This is not to suggest that exercise is some type of magic bullet, nor that exercise in and of itself can take the place of medicine. But regular exercise plays an irreplaceable role in the process of pre-habilitation, rehabilitation and post-habilitation. The goal is to find the proper dose of exercise to get the ideal response. It's important to remember that more is not always better, and what's good for one person is not right for another. This concept is not unlike trying to find the correct prescription of medication. The key is to train, not strain, and to have a program that is unique to you.

In Part 3 you'll find some corrective and preventive exercise to keep the hip healthy and functional. In addition, following the general guidelines below can dramatically reduce (re)injury:

- Avoid any exercise that allows you to bring your knee higher than 90 degrees towards your chest.
- Avoid repeated impact and heavy loads.
- If you're overweight, lose weight.
- Be careful when pivoting on your leg; move your whole body if possible.
- Avoid swinging your leg across the midline of your body or swinging it too far to the side.
- Don't do exaggerated leg movements in any position.
- Don't force any stretch or movement beyond your comfortable range of motion.
- When using resistance devices, you control the weight—don't let the weight control you.

Posture's Role in Prevention

Proper posture is essential in preventing injury and muscle imbalances. The interplay of the kinetic chain—what happens above or below the hip—can affect the hip joint. Experts now understand that if one body part

PROPER POSTURE CHECKLIST

- Stand with your weight over the balls of your feet and heels.
- Tuck your tailbone between your legs (imagine that you're resting on the edge of a bar stool) and make the distance from your belly button and your chest as far apart as possible; pull your belly button in.
- Place an imaginary apple under your chin.
- From a side view, your ears, shoulders and hips should be aligned. A mental picture that works for my students is to think of your body as a tube of toothpaste with all the forces squeezing you in and upright.
- When sitting, keep your ears aligned over your shoulders and your shoulders aligned over your hips; your knees are aligned over your ankles.

is misaligned, overused or hurt, it can affect the mechanics somewhere along the kinetic chain. For example, a simple sprained ankle that causes you to limp for a few days can throw your hip off, just as having a sway back and regularly locking out your knees can do the same thing.

How a person stands or moves will have a significant impact on his or her body alignment. For instance, sitting in a chair and leaning slightly to one side all day will affect the structure both above and below the hips or place unequal pressure on one side of the body. Finding correct alignment is far more difficult than you might think. Sure, you might be able to maintain correct balance while standing in a static position, but can you do it while jogging or doing chores? This is where body re-education comes in.

Keep in mind that decreased flexibility of the hip flexors, hamstrings and quadriceps can also contribute to hip dysfunction. This is often seen in people who are very active but either don't stretch or don't strengthen the opposing muscle group; they become more inflexible, thus compounding the problems they may already have. However, too much stretching can compromise the stability of the hip joint; overly lax joints can be just as bad as overly tight muscles. Think balance and symmetry.

High-Risk Areas

It helps to know the areas of the body that are vulnerable to injury. Besides the hips, the knees, neck, low back, shoulders and ankles are high-risk. Pay special attention when performing exercises that involve these areas, and follow these rules.

- Don't allow your legs to spread too wide or too far forward or back.
- Always perform exercises with proper execution.
- Don't neglect the small supporting actors of your hip joint (most of us focus on the "show" muscles and forget the importance of these smaller muscles).
- Pay attention to how your head, upper back and legs are positioned during activities of daily living and in the workplace.

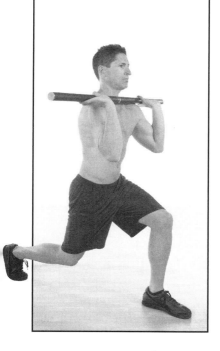

designing a hip routine

Research shows that most of the things that cause disease and dysfunction can be positively influenced by proper exercise, which can serve as a protective measure or a restorative tool. Hippocrates knew this as far back as 370 BC. He is known to have said, "Generally speaking, all parts of the body which have function, if used in moderation and exercised in labors to which each is accustomed, become healthy and well developed and age slowly. But if unused and left idle become liable to disease, defective in growth and age quickly." Or, said another way, "Use it or lose it!"

Corrective exercise has a positive influence on the majority of the body's tissues, organs and systems, and has several functions. It's useful in preventing, alleviating or curing a condition. Designing a therapeutic exercise program that will allow you to train at optimal levels requires either trial and error or skill and knowledge. The purpose of this section is to help you avoid the trial and error part.

One expert stated that at least 90 percent of exercise programs include some exercises that are as detrimental as they are valuable. When determining if an exercise is good for your body, ask yourself the following questions:
- Why am I doing this exercise/activity?
- What are the benefits of this exercise/activity?
- What are the risks of this exercise/activity?

- How do I feel while doing this exercise/activity?
- How do I feel after doing this exercise/activity?
- Does the activity work the targeted muscle?
- Could I receive the same benefits doing a different exercise/activity?

If an exercise/sport/activity fails the above criteria, look for another activity. Any exercise that makes it into your routine should

HEALTHY HIP TRAINING TIPS

- Identify and address a problem early; this keeps small problems small.
- Avoid over-training— balance your volume of training with your intensity of training.
- Allow your body to rest and recuperate.
- Learn your hip's safe range of motion. Each of us has a unique range of motion—one person's range may be another person's strain.
- Cross-train to prevent overuse syndrome; include exercises that train the small supporting muscles of your hip.
- Understand the possible dangers of too many ballistic and explosive movements in your activity.
- Train smart NOT heavy. Too much weight combined with poor execution equals injury! Any abuse of your body today may haunt you later in life
- Understand how to mix "reps" & "sets" for maximum gain and minimum risk.
- Learn how to prepare for activity, whether it be pre-season conditioning or pre-game joint readiness.
- Adapt your training by including plyometrics, periodization, and open-kinetic vs. closed-kinetic chain moves.

provide maximum return on investment. If your trainer fails to be mindful of the above considerations, find a different trainer.

Part 3 provides a fairly comprehensive collection of exercises that can be done around the hip joint. Some exercises, such as jumping exercises (plyometrics), should be used judiciously, while exercises such as standing leg raises can be performed regularly. The exercises for the most part are listed by the position from which they're performed: standing, seated, lying down. Generally, the most passive and gentle exercises are listed first.

When selecting an exercise, test-drive it a few times; see how it feels while you do it and, more importantly, how you feel after doing it. Any exercise selected should not make you feel worse. The simple key is to determine how you feel two hours post-exercise. Never load up on medications prior to exercise to mask your pain.

Note: Prior to performing any exercise, it is strongly suggested that you warm up your hip joint. Some people enjoy a warm shower or bath; others gently ride a stationary bike before performing the exercises.

As for how many you should do? It's an individual thing. I find it interesting that everybody wants to be considered unique, but when it comes to exercise, they want to do what the person next to them is doing. Remember why you purchased this book—

you had a hip concern, so approach every exercise cautiously.

However, as a general guideline, start out with 3–5 repetitions (reps) while listening to your body. Wait a day and see how you feel. Select only one or two exercises to start with and see how you feel afterward. If you select ten exercises and do them all, you won't know which one caused the ill effect. Eventually, your goal will be 2 sets of 10 reps of each exercise. Change exercises every three to four weeks and increase resistance when it feels effortless.

Don't become complacent about exercise. It's critical that you be mindful of proper body mechanics when working out and associate with your body while working out. This means pay attention to what you're doing. Remember that only perfect practice makes perfect. You might consider not listening to music while exercising because it's hard to stay focused while doing so. It's also wise to have your equipment adjusted correctly for you; a bike seat that's too high can contribute to pelvic issues, and running shoes that are worn can cause problems as well.

Change your routine periodically. This allows your body to adapt to something different and to use muscles differently, which prevents overuse syndrome and keeps your efforts from becoming stale. One method to try is periodization. These techniques may be incorporated to train the body in a different cycle. Continuing to do the same workout in the same order will lead to boredom and possible overuse injury.

Here are some ways to vary your routine:

- Change/vary the *frequency* of the workout.
- Change/vary the *intensity* of the workout, within reason.
- Change/vary the *time* of your workouts.
- Change/vary the *type* of exercise you do by cross-training.
- Change/vary the *rest period* between intervals.

- Combine multiple movements simultaneously in an exercise.

Controversial Exercises

It's been well documented that regular exercise and physical activity are good for the body. Unfortunately, sometimes we hurt ourselves by following outdated principles or faulty assumptions. This section highlights some popular exercises that fail the "benefit-to-risk index" (that is, their risks outweigh their benefits), or exercises that may contribute to hip problems if performed incorrectly. By staying mindful of these common high-risk exercises, you reduce your chances of injury. Most of the following won't kill you today or even really hurt you

if done once or twice. The problem is cumulative—they manifest themselves over time.

1. *Leg presses*—Being too close can cramp your range of motion and place undue stress on your hip joint when pressing the weight out.

2. *Full squats*—Squatting down past 90 degrees with a weight across your shoulders can contribute to major hip problems down the road.

3. *Explosive plyometric moves*—While good for sports training, these are actually bad for life. Jumping onto a box or over a bar to improve explosive power may contribute to hip issues later in life.

4. *Deep lunges/wide dynamic jumping jacks or dance moves*—

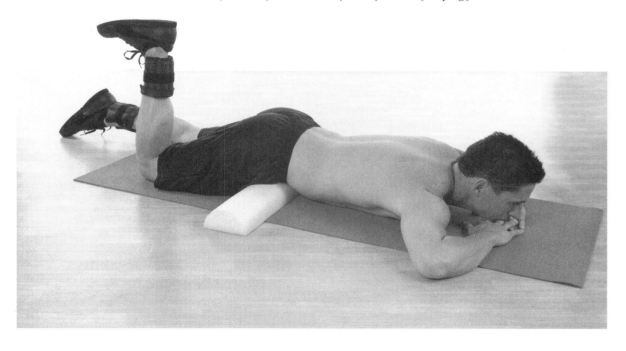

Allowing your knees to wobble or go past your toes can transfer excessive force to the hip and pelvic region.

5. *Running/jumping bleacher stairs*—This places tremendous loads onto the hip area. Jumping down is especially bad for the hip joint.

6. *Cycling*— Poor biomechanics (i.e., chronic misuse) will result in hip dysfunction further down the road.

7. *Running*—Poor biomechanics (i.e., chronic misuse) will result in hip dysfunction further down the road.

8. *Rowing*—Using improper leg alignment will add to hip dysfunction.

9. *Extreme high-impact activities such as parachuting or bungee jumping*—Sudden impacts can jar the hip joint.

Note: Any water exercise equipment or movements that replicate contraindicated exercises are to be avoided. While water is an excellent place to exercise, poor biomechanics and classes taught by ill-trained instructors can hurt you. In addition, any activity/sport that places you at risk for a fall or impact (such as ice skating, football or skateboarding) can contribute to a hip problem; it might be wise to wear hip protection.

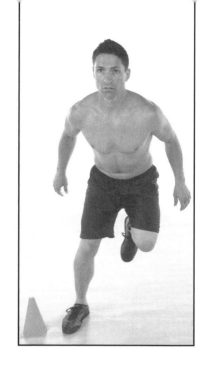

sample conditioning programs

This section features hip programs for several common hip conditions and sports/activities. It also includes a program for general overall conditioning. Assuming you are pain-free and have received clearance from your doctor, locate the program that applies to you and perform it daily; a cross-training approach in which you stretch daily and do the conditioning exercises 2–3 times a week might work well.

If an exercise does not feel right, ask yourself the questions on page 31 to determine if you should remove the exercise from your routine.

Prior to doing any exercise, remember to warm up the joint area. A warm-up is not the same as stretching—a warm-up is simply any activity that increases muscle temperature so the joint is more limber. Tight muscles,

ligaments and tendons are more inclined to be injured.

Determining how long to hold a stretch or how many reps to do is truly an individual decision. There is no magic formula that will work for everyone; each person will respond differently. Avoid overdoing it; more is not always better. The bottom line is your hip will tell you how far to stretch and how long to hold

it. However, if you don't have an existing hip issue, you can follow the basic protocol noted on page 32. Some of the programs will suggest strengthening exercises that utilize a band or a dumbbell. If you have one but not the other, feel free to do the exercise with the prop that's available. Stability ball exercises can often be done on the floor as well.

general conditioning

This program is for people with no hip issues, focusing on improving stability of the hip region, strengthening the area, and fostering better flexibility.

STRETCH

	PAGE	EXERCISE
	53	Sit & Reach
	65	Butterfly
	61	Standing Hip Flexor
	59	Rear Calf Stretch

ACTIVE EXERCISE

	PAGE	EXERCISE
	69	Knee to Chest
	72	Standing Leg Extension
	93	Side-Lying Leg Lift
	94	Reverse Side-Lying Leg Lift
	96	Clam
	97	Prone Leg Curl
	106	Pelvic Lift on Ball
	75	Lunge
	83	Bike Ride
	100	Bicycle
	112	Superman Prone

arthritis

While curing arthritis is difficult, sensible management is paramount. Too often many people with arthritis stop moving, which causes further stiffness and muscle weakness.

STRETCH

	PAGE	EXERCISE
	50	Seated Knee to Chest
	51	Single Knee to Chest
	53	Sit & Reach

ACTIVE EXERCISE

	PAGE	EXERCISE
	73	Straight-Leg Lift
	87	Leg Squeeze & Spread
	89	Quad Setting
	92	Hip Tilt & Roll
	118	Ball Bicycle
	93	Side-Lying Leg Lift
	94	Reverse Side-Lying Leg Lift

groin strain

The healing process of a groin strain is painfully slow. If available, water rehab, from gentle leg exercises to light jogging and flutter kicking in the pool, is quite helpful. The goal is to foster healing and prevent scar tissue. Speak to your health provider about performing ice massage to that area. Prior to exercising, warm up the area and engage in gentle stretching after given permission from doctor.

STRETCH

	PAGE	EXERCISE
	51	Single Knee to Chest
	52	Double Knee to Chest
	57	Hamstrings Grab
	61	Standing Hip Flexor
	65	Butterfly
	66	Outer Thigh Stretch
	24	Foam Roller Hamstrings

ACTIVE EXERCISE

	PAGE	EXERCISE
	70	Weight Shift
	72	Standing Leg Extension
	85	Side-Step
	87	Leg Squeeze & Spread
	94	Reverse Side-Lying Leg Lift
	95	Rotate Leg In & Out
	96	Clam
	125	Side-to-Side Hop

osteoporosis

Osteoporosis is a serious bone-loss condition that frequently involves the hip region. When doing hip exercises, consult your doctor for any precautions. The key here is to strengthen the hip area while not placing too much load on the joint to cause a fracture. Keep in mind the robustness of the bone is related to the forces applied to it. Use caution when performing stretches; don't force the moves. Besides performing the exercises listed, walking with a weighted vest can be helpful.

Precautions

- Avoid any rapid twisting motions
- Avoid pivoting with one foot planted
- Avoid heavy impact activities
- Avoid heavy squats

STRETCH

	PAGE	EXERCISE
	61	Standing Hip Flexor
	59	Rear Calf Stretch

ACTIVE EXERCISE

	PAGE	EXERCISE
	72	Standing Leg Extension
	73	Straight-Leg Lift
	75	Lunge (with caution)
	89	Quad Setting
	79	Transition to Standing
	86	Sit to Stand
	106	Pelvic Lift on Ball

baseball & softball

Whether played casually or at a competitive level, baseball and softball require a lot of standing that places a load on the hip region.

STRETCH

	PAGE	EXERCISE
	50	Seated Knee to Chest
	52	Double Knee to Chest
	54	Crossed-Leg Drop
	57	Hamstrings Grab
	59	Rear Calf Stretch
	67	Ankle Circle

ACTIVE EXERCISE

	PAGE	EXERCISE
	115	Ball Squat
	78	Side Lunge
	70	Weight Shift
	74	Standing Leg Curl
	75	Lunge
	77	Lunge & Twist
	105	Side Plank
	110	Prone Leg Lift

biking

Regardless of whether you bike casually or seriously, bicycling too long or too hard can cause injury and muscle imbalances. To prevent problems, make sure your bike seat is adjusted correctly forward and aft. Also, learning to use the gears correctly to "spin" is better on the hips than "grinding" at lower RPMs. If you're a serious cyclist, engaging in regular upper body conditioning may help your climbing ability.

STRETCH

	PAGE	EXERCISE
	51	Single Knee to Chest
	60	Quad Stretch
	62	Kneeling Hip Flexor
	64	Piriformis Stretch
	59	Rear Calf Stretch
	67	Ankle Circle

ACTIVE EXERCISE

	PAGE	EXERCISE
	73	Straight-Leg Lift
	74	Standing Leg Curl
	76	Lunge with Bar
	80	Squat with Dumbbell
	91	Gas Pedal
	109	Ball Roll-Out

bowling

While some people might not consider bowling a sport, its asymmetrical and explosive nature can be very hard on the hip and lower back. Always warm up the body prior to going full steam ahead.

STRETCH

	PAGE	EXERCISE
	53	Sit & Reach
	61	Standing Hip Flexor
	59	Rear Calf Stretch

ACTIVE EXERCISE

	PAGE	EXERCISE
	80	Squat with Dumbbell
	75	Lunge
	72	Standing Leg Extension
	82	Single-Leg Squat

field sports

Soccer, football, field hockey and lacrosse require a great deal of running and pivoting on an uneven field, which can be problematic for the hip.

STRETCH

	PAGE	EXERCISE
	52	Double Knee to Chest
	54	Crossed-Leg Drop
	55	Figure 4
	56	Inverted Figure 4
	57	Hamstrings Grab
	58	TFL Stretch
	59	Rear Calf Stretch
	60	Quad Stretch
	62	Kneeling Hip Flexor
	64	Piriformis Stretch
	65	Butterfly

ACTIVE EXERCISE

	PAGE	EXERCISE
	119	Forward/Backward Jump & Hold
	120	Lateral Jump & Hold
	121	One-Leg Hop & Hold
	122	Speed Play: Hard/Easy
	123	Lateral Shuffle
	124	Circle Jump
	125	Side-to-Side Hop
	126	Double-Leg Jump

golf

While golf looks effortless, it can be very hard on the hips and lower back. Since golf is repetitive, the worse a player you are, the more repetitive it is. It helps to have a strong core and stable hip platform.

jogging/running

Most joggers/runners train for their activity by doing more of the same, setting them up for injury. Each time a person jogs, the forces placed on the lower extremities is significant, with much of the load transferred to the hip. Cross-training with water exercise, deep-water running or biking is a wise idea, as is sometimes even resting. While this routine will not improve race times, it can keep you doing what you enjoy. Keep in mind that if you're a runner, you may have muscle imbalances—so stretch what is tight and strengthen what is lax.

STRETCH

ACTIVE EXERCISE

racquet sports

Tennis and racquetball are popular sports that can be played at many levels, but they require quick moves and jarring impact, which over time can have a significant effect on the hip joint.

STRETCH

	PAGE	EXERCISE
	52	Double Knee to Chest
	64	Piriformis Stretch
	65	Butterfly
	61	Standing Hip Flexor

ACTIVE EXERCISE

	PAGE	EXERCISE
	102	Pelvic Lift
	78	Side Lunge
	72	Standing Leg Extension
	120	Lateral Jump & Hold
	119	Forward/Backward Jump & Hold
	127	Single-Leg Hop
	107	Bridge on Ball
	111	Double-Leg Lift

skiing (downhill)

Downhill skiing is a vigorous sport done in cold weather that involves a great deal of turning and impact when going over the "bump." All of these variables set up the skier for injury, thereby increasing the necessity that you be well conditioned to participate. This routine focuses on joint preparation; it is advised that you prepare the hips, knee and back for all the impacts and twists.

STRETCH

	PAGE	EXERCISE
	67	Ankle Circle
	61	Standing Hip Flexor
	59	Rear Calf Stretch
	65	Butterfly

ACTIVE EXERCISE

	PAGE	EXERCISE
	72	Standing Leg Extension
	73	Straight-Leg Lift
	74	Standing Leg Curl
	77	Lunge & Twist
	78	Side Lunge
	81	Downhill Skier
	82	Single-Leg Squat
	89	Quad Setting
	108	Leg Extension on Ball
	113	Pointer Series
	115	Ball Squat
	119	Forward/Backward Jump & Hold
	120	Lateral Jump & Hold
	121	One-Leg Hop & Hold
	124	Circle Jump
	126	Double-Leg Jump

skiing (cross-country)

From a physiological point of view, cross-country skiing is one of the most physically demanding sports yet can be done at different levels, from a slow cruise through the woods to a extremely challenging run. It can require great muscular and cardiovascular endurance as well as flexibility, so it's wise to train to play, not just show up on the hill unconditioned, which can lead to injury.

STRETCH

PAGE	EXERCISE
54	Crossed-Leg Drop
55	Figure 4
57	Hamstrings Grab
59	Rear Calf Stretch
60	Quad Stretch

ACTIVE EXERCISE

PAGE	EXERCISE
68	Knee Lift
72	Standing Leg Extension
75	Lunge
82	Single-Leg Squat
83	Bike Ride
85	Side-Step
87	Leg Squeeze & Spread
89	Quad Setting
91	Gas Pedal
93	Side-Lying Leg Lift
94	Reverse Side-Lying Leg Lift
95	Rotate Leg In & Out
98	Hands & Knees Leg Curl
112	Superman Prone
115	Ball Squat

part 3

the
exercises

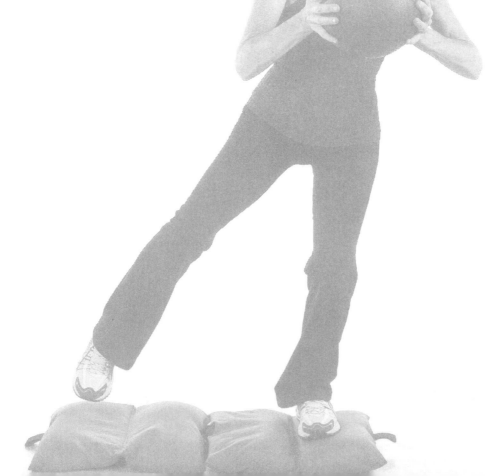

50

stretches
seated knee to chest
lower back, gluteus maximus

CAUTION: If you have osteoporosis/osteopenia, do not pull your knees in past 90 degrees.

STARTING POSITION: Sit with proper posture in a stable chair and place your feet on the floor.

starting position

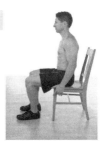

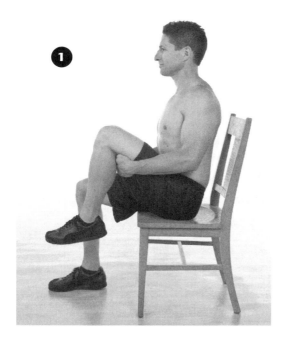

1 Clasp both hands beneath your left leg and bring your left knee toward your chest. Hold this position for a comfortable moment, feeling the stretch in the gluteal region.

Release the knee, switch sides and repeat.

CAUTION: *If you have osteoporosis/osteopenia, do not pull your knees in past 90 degrees.*

STARTING POSITION: Lie on a mat and, if needed, place a pillow under your head. You may want to weigh down your non-lifting leg with an ankle weight on the thigh.

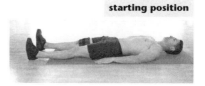

starting position

1 Clasp behind your free thigh with both hands and gently pull your knee to your chest. Hold this position for a comfortable moment, feeling the stretch in your bottom and low back.

Return to starting position and switch sides.

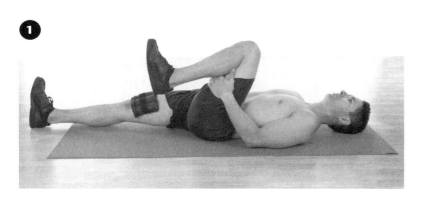

VARIATION: For an additional stretch in your straight-leg hip flexor, you can also try this by lying on a higher surface, such as a weight bench.

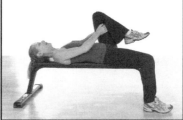

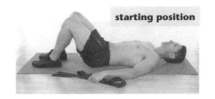

starting position

CAUTION: If you have osteoporosis/osteopenia, do not pull your knees in past 90 degrees.

STARTING POSITION: Lie on a mat and, if needed, place a pillow under your head. Bend your knees and place both feet flat on the floor.

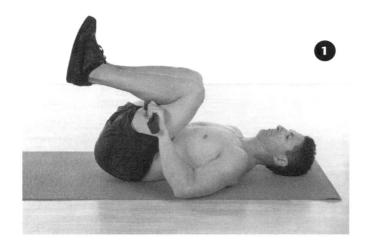

1

1 Loop a strap behind the backs of both legs and hold an end of the strap in each hand. Gently pull the straps to bring your knees to your chest. Hold this position for a comfortable moment, feeling the stretch in your bottom and low back.

VARIATION: Use just your hands to draw in your knees.

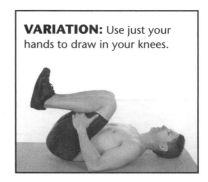

CAUTION: Be careful not to tip the chair over.

STARTING POSITION: Sit at the edge of a stable chair. Loop a strap around the ball of your left foot and hold an end of the strap in each hand. Extend your legs straight out in front of you and place your heels on the floor with your toes pointing up close to 90 degrees.

starting position

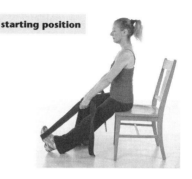

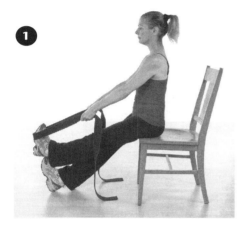

1 Stack your left heel on top of your right foot, keeping your legs as straight as possible. Inhale deeply through your nose.

2 Exhale through your lips and gently pull yourself forward by leading with your chest rather than rounding your back.

Switch sides and repeat.

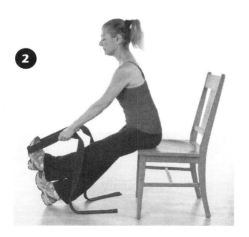

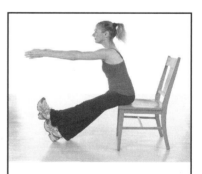

INTERMEDIATE: Instead of using the strap, you can extend your arms forward and gently reach forward with your fingertips.

ADVANCED: Place both heels on a chair in front of you.

POSITION: Lie on your side on the edge of a bed or bench. Be careful not to roll off. Gently allow the top leg to drop off the side as far as is comfortable. Breathe into the stretch and relax. Hold for 10–30 seconds, as tolerated.

Repeat 3–5 times, then switch sides.

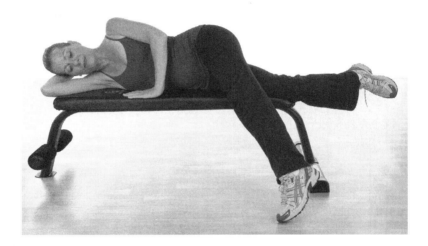

figure 4

hamstrings, lower back

55

CAUTION: Avoid this move if you have knee problems.

STARTING POSITION: Sit on a mat with both legs extended straight out in front of you. Keep your torso as tall as possible.

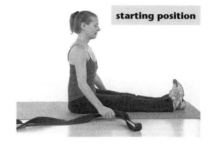
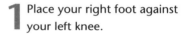

starting position

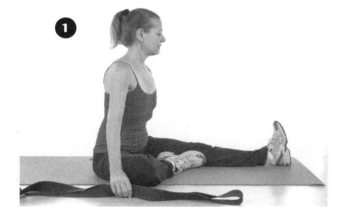

1 Place your right foot against your left knee.

2 Loop a strap around the sole of your left foot and hold on to the ends of the strap. Inhale deeply through your nose. While keeping your head and torso tall, pull yourself forward until you feel a comfortable stretch in the backs of your legs. Hold this stretch for a comfortable moment, focusing on the sensation of the stretch, not on going as far as possible. The goal is to hold the stretch for 60 seconds. Exhale and return to the starting position.

Switch sides and repeat.

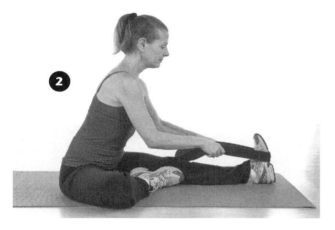

CAUTION: If you have osteoporosis/osteopenia, do not pull your knees in past 90 degrees.

STARTING POSITION: Lie on a mat with your knees bent and your feet flat on the floor.

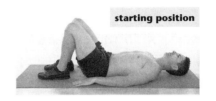

starting position

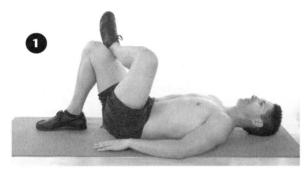

1 Place your left ankle on top of your right knee. Inhale deeply through your nose.

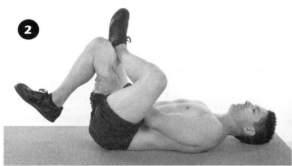

2 Wrap both hands around your right leg and bring your knee and ankle to your chest while exhaling.

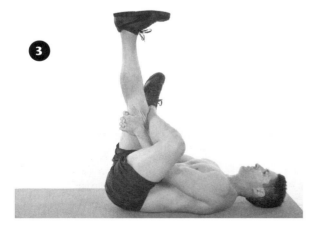

3 Now straighten your right leg toward the ceiling as much as is comfortable. Focus on inhaling and exhaling fully and hold this stretch.

Switch sides and repeat.

STARTING POSITION: Lie on your back with your knees bent and feet flat on the floor.

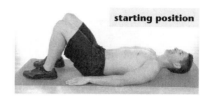

starting position

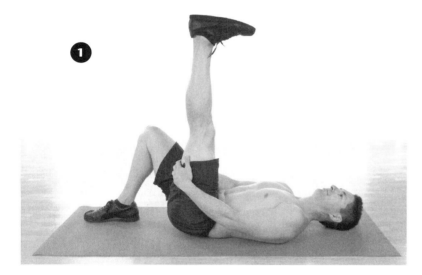

1 Grab the back of your left leg, above or below the knee, and pull your leg toward your chest, keeping your leg slightly bent. Attempt to comfortably straighten your leg toward the ceiling. Hold for 10–30 seconds, as tolerated.

Return to starting position then switch sides. Repeat twice on each side.

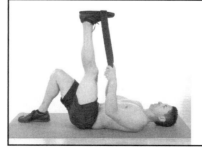

MODIFICATION: Loop a strap around the ball of the foot before extending the leg toward the ceiling.

VARIATION: If you have a flexible back and hamstrings, you can also straighten the leg that's on the floor.

Caution: If you've had hip replacement surgery, take extra care when doing this. If you have osteoporosis/osteopenia, do not pull your knees in past 90 degrees.

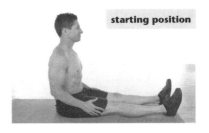

starting position

STARTING POSITION: Sit upright on the floor with your legs out in front of you. Maintain good posture.

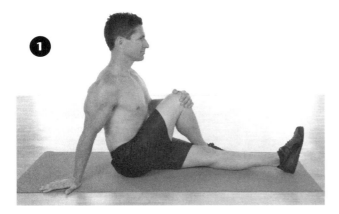

1

1 Cross your right leg over your left thigh and tuck your left foot by your right buttock.

2 Exhale as you place your left elbow on the outside of your right thigh and gently twist your upper body to the right. Hold for 15 seconds.

Switch sides and repeat.

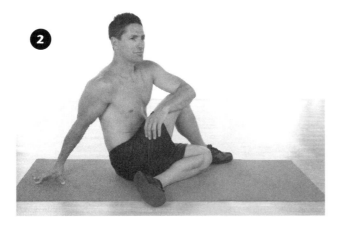

2

VARIATION: This can also be done with the bottom leg extended.

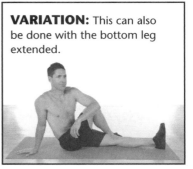

STARTING POSITION: Stand behind a chair, placing both hands on the back of the chair.

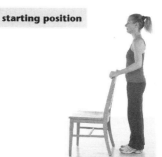

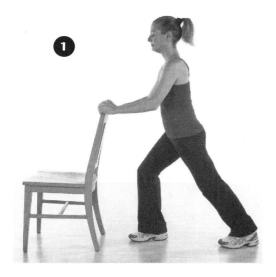

1 Keeping the heel down, slide your left leg as far back as you can.

Bend your left knee until the desired stretch is felt in the calf area. Hold this stretch for a comfortable moment.

Switch sides and repeat.

CAUTION: *Avoid this exercise if you have poor balance. STOP if you notice undue compression in your knee or experience any low back discomfort. If you feel a cramp coming on, do a hamstrings stretch.*

STARTING POSITION: Stand with proper posture facing a chair.

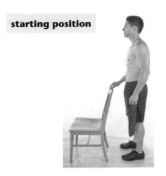

starting position

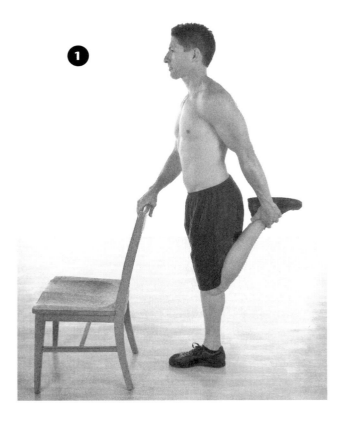

1 Grab your left ankle with your left hand and gently pull your left heel toward your bottom. Keep both knees as close together as possible. Use the back of a chair for balance if necessary. Hold this stretch for a comfortable moment.

Switch sides and repeat.

MODIFICATION: You may also loop a strap around your ankle if you can't reach your foot.

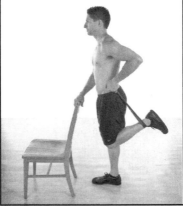

STARTING POSITION: Stand tall with proper posture.

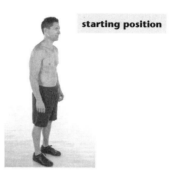

starting position

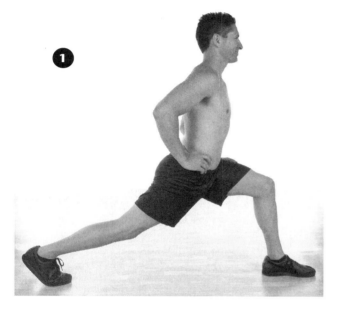

1 Slide your right leg back a comfortable distance. Pushing your rear heel toward the floor, gently tuck your tailbone under, press your hips forward and arch your back slightly. Hold this stretch for a comfortable moment, focusing on feeling the stretch in the upper leg/hip region rather than in the calf area.

Switch sides and repeat.

MODIFICATION: If balance is an issue, do this next to a chair or wall.

CAUTION: Avoid this stretch if you have poor balance and/or bad knees.

STARTING POSITION: Kneel on a mat or something soft to protect your knees.

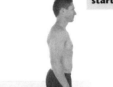

starting position

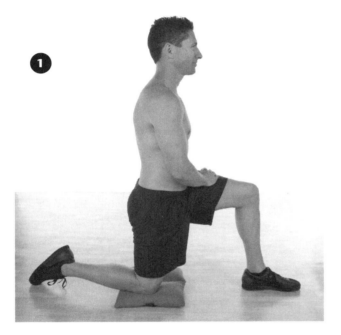

1 Move your left knee forward so that you can place your left foot flat on the floor. Maintain an erect position, lifting your chin, squeezing your shoulder blades together, pulling in your belly button and contracting your gluteals. Slowly press your hips forward until you feel a comfortable stretch in the front of your kneeling leg. Hold this stretch for a comfortable moment. Be aware of any cramping in the hamstring of the front leg.

MODIFICATION: If balance is an issue, do this next to a chair or wall.

STARTING POSITION: Rest on your hands and knees.

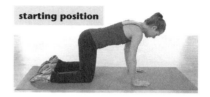

starting position

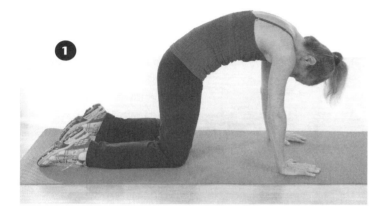

1 Draw your belly button in, causing your back to round. Inhale deeply.

2 Exhale and slowly relax your body to the starting position.

Repeat as desired.

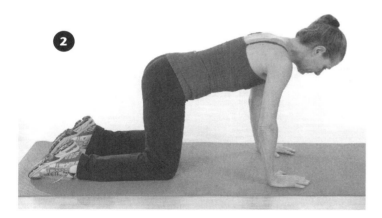

The piriformis muscle is a deep-lying muscle in the gluteal region, through which some believe the sciatic nerve passes. When the piriformis is too tight, it is believed to cramp the sciatic nerve, causing the symptoms of sciatica.

STARTING POSITION: Lie on a mat with your knees bent and your feet flat on the floor.

starting position

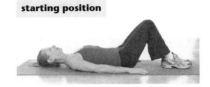

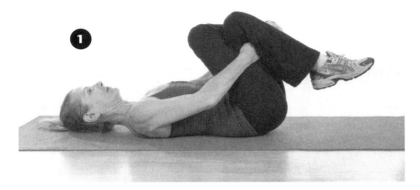

1 Cross your right knee on top of your left knee and grab behind your left leg with both hands. Gently pull your knees in toward your chest. Stop when tension occurs. Hold this position for a comfortable moment, focusing on the sensation of the stretch.

Switch sides and repeat.

MODIFICATION: Loop a strap around your lower leg if you can't reach.

STARTING POSITION: Sit on a mat with your knees bent and your feet flat on the floor. Place the soles of your feet together and gently allow your knees to drop to the floor.

starting position

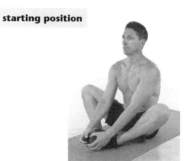

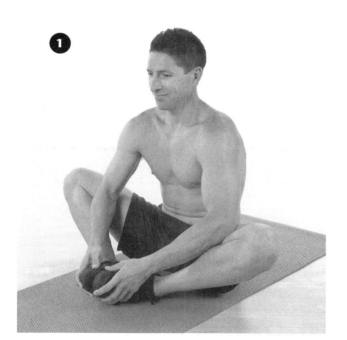

1 Use your forearms to apply gentle pressure to your thighs. Hold this stretch.

VARIATION: Use your hands to gently help your knees to the floor.

CAUTION: If you've been advised by your doctor or therapist not to cross your legs, do not do this exercise.

STARTING POSITION: Stand with proper posture next to a chair on your left side.

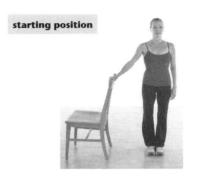

starting position

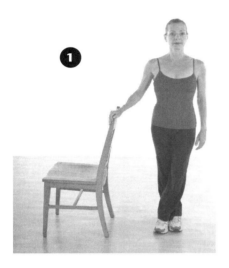

1 Cross your left leg in front of your right leg.

2 Raise your left arm up overhead and lean to the right, gently pressing your left hip outward to the left. Use the chair for balance. Hold this stretch.

Switch sides and repeat

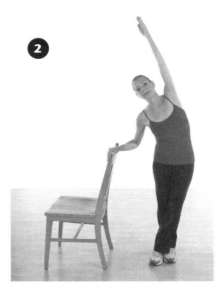

VARIATION: If your shoulders are tight, just place your hand on your hips.

ADVANCED: If balance is not an issue, try this without the chair.

STARTING POSITION: Sit at the edge of a stable chair.

starting position

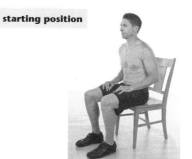

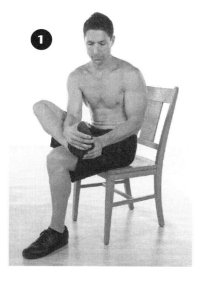

1 Cross your right ankle on top of your left knee and gently grasp your foot with your hands.

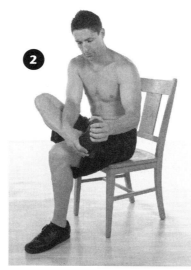

2–3 Slowly use your hands to gently move your foot in comfortable circles as well as forward and backward.

Switch sides and repeat.

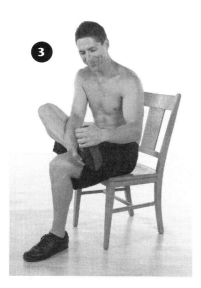

VARIATION: This can also be done without hands by straightening your leg in front of you and slowly circling your ankle in all directions.

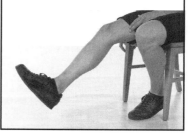

STARTING POSITION: Stand tall with good posture.

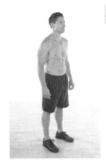

starting position

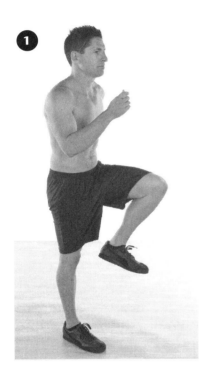

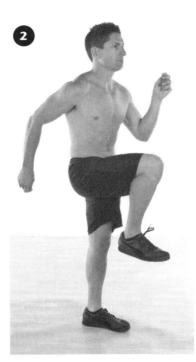

1–2 March in place, gradually lifting your knees higher as you warm up. As you limber up, swing your arms in opposition as you lift your knees.

Continue for 1–3 minutes or longer.

CAUTION: *If you don't have good balance, please perform this move while lying on your back (see page 51). If you have osteoporosis, do NOT lift your knee to hip level.*

STARTING POSITION: Stand tall with good posture.

starting position

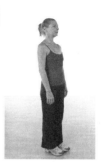

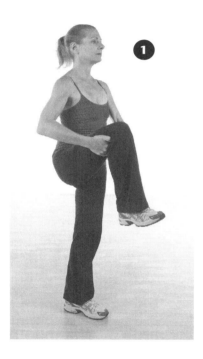

1 Lift your right leg up as high as is comfortable; reach around your leg/knee and hug it to your chest for 3–5 seconds.

Lower slowly to the starting position and switch sides. Continue performing this move for 1–2 minutes.

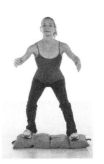

CAUTION: Do not do this if you have a history of falling.

STARTING POSITION: Stand tall on a soft foam pad with your feet shoulder-width apart and shoulders back. Maintain your balance for a few seconds.

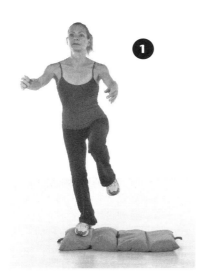

1-2 Once this becomes easy, shift your body weight to one foot; hold for 5 seconds.

Continue shifting your weight.

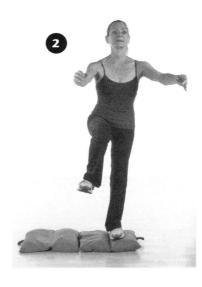

If you find this exercise too difficult, try it without weights.

STARTING POSITION: Strap an ankle weight around each ankle and stand with proper posture. Place your right hand on a stable chair for balance.

starting position

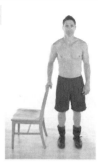

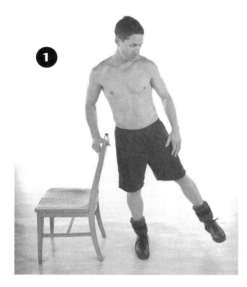

1 Keeping your foot pointed forward, slowly raise the outside leg out to the side as high as is comfortable and hold.

2 Slowly return to starting position with control.

Repeat, then switch sides.

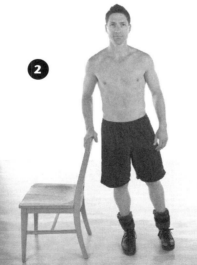

VARIATION: To perform this with an exercise band, tie the ends of the band together and loop it around both ankles.

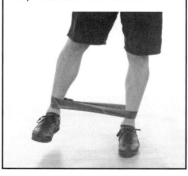

If you find this exercise too difficult, try it without weights.

STARTING POSITION: Strap an ankle weight around each ankle and stand with proper posture next to a sturdy chair. Hold onto the chair for balance if necessary.

starting position

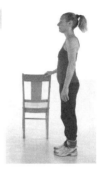

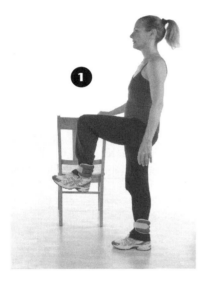

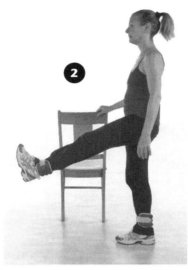

1 Lift your right thigh in front of you as high as is comfortable (but no higher than parallel with the floor).

2 Slowly extend (kick) your right foot forward until it is fully extended. Hold for a count of 1–2.

3 Slowly bend your knee.

Repeat, then switch sides.

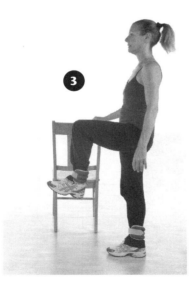

MODIFICATION: If you're not strong enough to hold the leg up unsupported, use your hands to help keep the leg up, but do not do this if you have poor balance.

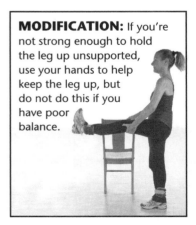

If you find this exercise too difficult, try it without weights.

STARTING POSITION: Strap an ankle weight around each ankle and stand to the left of a sturdy chair. Place your hand on the back of the chair for balance. Maintain proper posture throughout the movement.

starting position

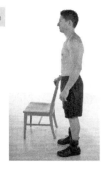

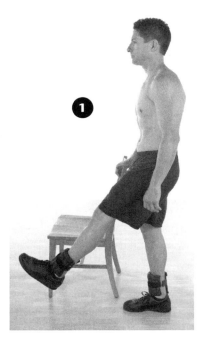

1 Keeping your outside leg straight, move it forward as high as is comfortable. Make sure you don't lean back while you raise your leg.

2 Slowly return to starting position.

Repeat, then switch sides.

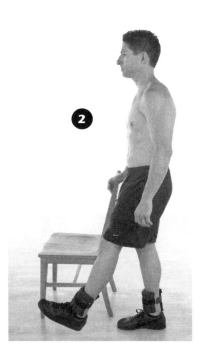

standing series
standing leg curl

If you find this exercise too difficult, try it without weights.

CAUTION: Avoid this exercise if you have lower back issues.

STARTING POSITION: Strap an ankle weight around each ankle and stand with proper posture, both feet together. Hold on to the back of a stable chair for balance.

starting position

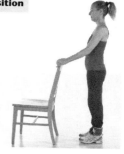

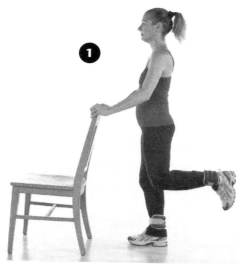

1 Slowly curl your left leg up toward your buttocks. Stop when your leg is parallel to the ground.

2 Hold for a moment, then slowly return the leg to starting position.

Repeat, then switch sides.

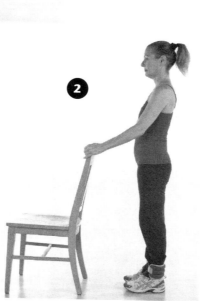

If you find this exercise too difficult, do this without weights and place your hands on your hips instead.

STARTING POSITION: Stand with proper posture and hold a dumbbell in each hand by your sides.

starting position

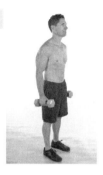

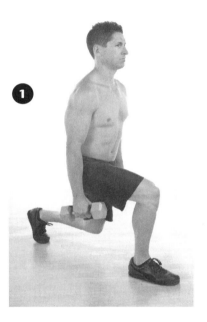

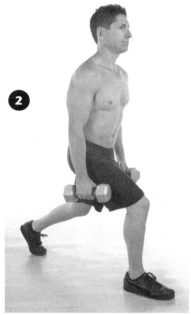

1 Keeping your left leg in place, lunge forward with your right leg as far as is comfortable, but keeping your knee in line with your ankle.

2 Step back to starting position.

Repeat, then switch sides.

MODIFICATION: If balance is an issue, hold a dumbbell in one hand and hold onto a chair with your free hand.

VARIATION: As your balance and strength improve, alternate legs with each lunge rather than doing all reps on one side.

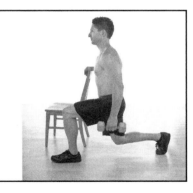

STARTING POSITION: Stand with proper posture and a body bar held across your chest, palms face-up.

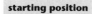

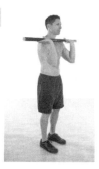

starting position

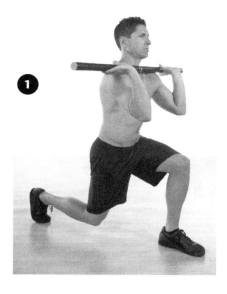

1 Lunge forward with your left leg as far as is comfortable, but keep your front knee in line with your ankle.

Step back to starting position. Switch sides.

CAUTION: If you have back issues, do not do this exercise.

STARTING POSITION: Stand tall with good posture, holding a weight or medicine ball straight out in front of you.

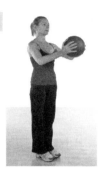

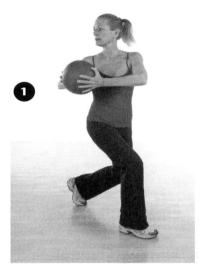

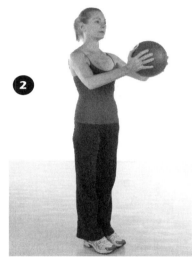

1 With your right leg, step forward a comfortable distance and twist slowly to the right.

2 Return to starting position.

3 Step forward with your left leg while slowly twisting to the left.

Continue alternating legs.

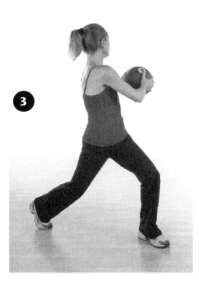

STARTING POSITION: Stand tall with good posture and hold a medicine ball in front of your chest.

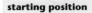

starting position

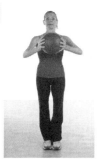

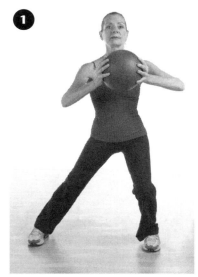

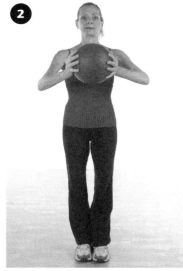

1 Step your right foot out to the side and bend your knee, keeping it behind your toes.

2 Return to starting position.

3 Step your left foot out to the side.

Continue for 1–3 minutes or longer.

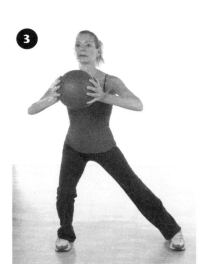

MODIFICATION: This can also be done without a medicine ball.

The strength of your legs is critical to your functional ability. Often when our hip hurts, we compensate and place undue stress on the hip, the lower back and/or the knees. Thus learning to get up mindfully will prevent further pain and trauma. Before you try to do regular squats, you need to learn to transition from sitting to standing correctly and put that information into muscle memory for daily use.

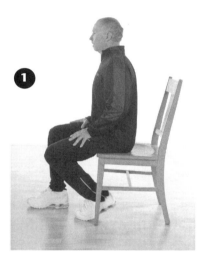

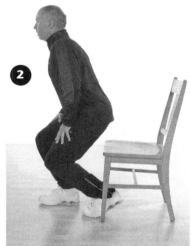

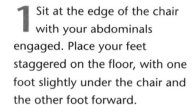

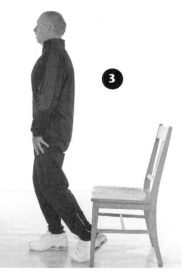

1 Sit at the edge of the chair with your abdominals engaged. Place your feet staggered on the floor, with one foot slightly under the chair and the other foot forward.

2 Start the movement from your pelvis area, rolling forward off your rear end and transferring your weight to your heels.

3 Press your weight into the floor, starting with putting weight into your heels, then roll forward using your momentum to assist you to a standing position.

Repeat, alternating the leg that's forward if possible.

VARIATION: If you have trouble with the staggered-feet option, try placing both feet slightly under the chair before standing.

Squats foster greater leg strength and provide stabilization to compromised knee joints.

STARTING POSITION: Stand tall with your feet shoulder-width apart. Hold one dumbbell with both hands, letting your arms hang in front of you.

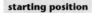

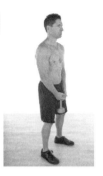

starting position

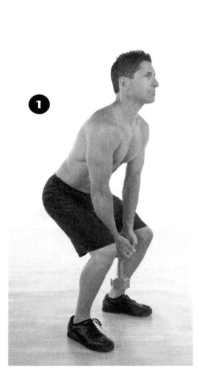

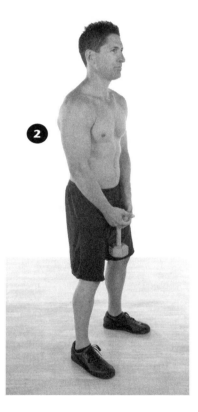

1 Keeping your back in neutral spine position, bend your knees to lower your rear end into a half-squat. Make sure your knees stay behind your toes.

2 Return to starting position.

MODIFICATION: For more support, you can sit into a chair and then get up.

If you find this exercise too difficult, try it without weights.

STARTING POSITION: Stand with both feet as close together as is comfortable, holding a weight or medicine ball in front of your chest.

starting position

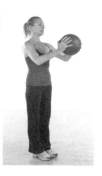

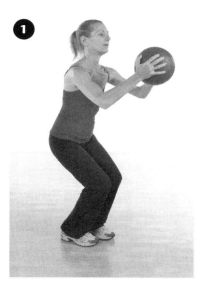

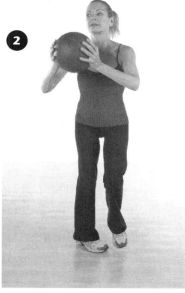

1 Squat down a quarter of the way, keeping your feet flat on the floor and your knees over your toes. Do not allow your knees to turn in or out. Hold for a count of 1–2–3–4–5.

2–3 As if skiing, flow through the starting position to perform a quarter-squat 45 degrees to the other side.

Continue switching sides.

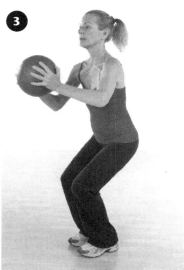

MODIFICATION: If balance is an issue, try the movement without weights and hold onto a chair for support.

If you find this exercise too difficult, try it without weights.

STARTING POSITION: Stand tall with proper posture.

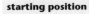
starting position

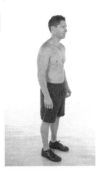

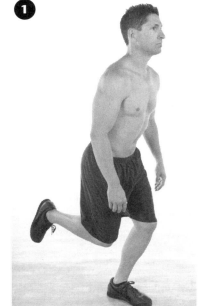

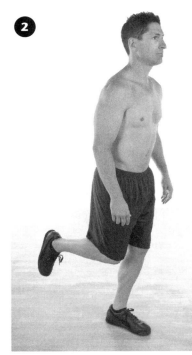

1 Bring your right heel up halfway toward your buttocks or as high as is comfortable, then slowly squat down as low as you can on your other leg, keeping your foot flat on the floor.

2 Slowly return to full standing position.

Repeat, then switch sides.

MODIFICATION: If balance is an issue, hold onto a chair or wall with one hand for support.

VARIATION: You can also do this with a dumbbell in each hand.

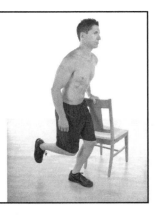

CAUTION: Do not do this if you have a history of falling.

STARTING POSITION: Stand tall with your feet shoulder-width apart and shoulders back. Hold your arms in front of you as if grasping handlebars.

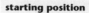
starting position

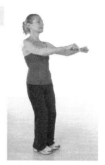

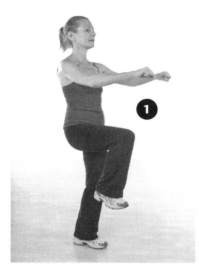

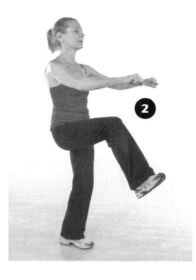

1–3 Shift your weight to your left leg and lift your right leg. Pretend that you are riding a bike with only one pedal.

Continue for the recommended time, maintaining proper form.

Rest then repeat with your other leg.

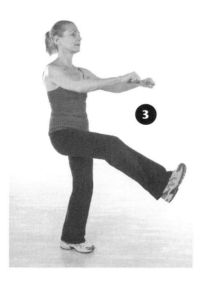

CAUTION: *If you experience any knee joint discomfort or swelling, discontinue this exercise.*

STARTING POSITION: Stand tall facing a sturdy bench, step or staircase. Make sure to hold onto something if you have poor balance.

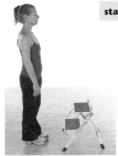

starting position

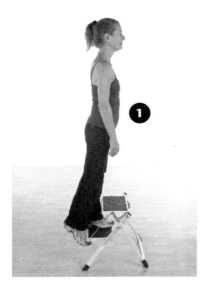

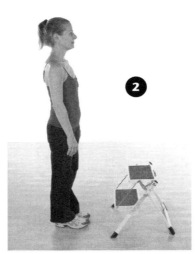

1 Step your left foot onto the step. Make sure your kneecap does not angle to the left or right when stepping, and keep your knee behind your big toe.

2 Return to starting position.

3 Step your right foot onto the step.

Continue alternating legs.

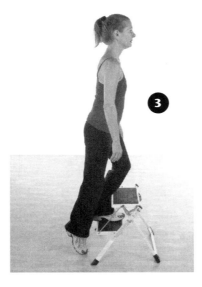

MODIFICATION: As your strength increases, you can increase the height of the step, hold a dumbbell in both hands or wear a weighted vest.

STARTING POSITION: Stand with the left side of your body next to a sturdy bench, step or staircase.

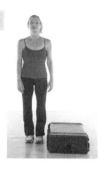

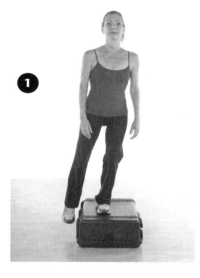

1 Step your left foot onto the step, leaving enough room for your right foot.

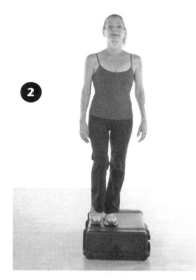

2 Step your right foot next to your left.

3 Step down with your right foot.

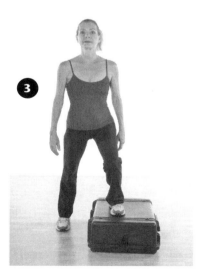

4 Step down with your left foot.

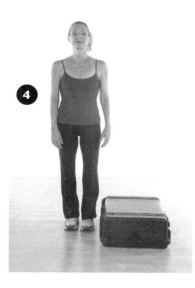

Repeat by standing with your right side to the step.

STARTING POSITION: Sit toward the front of a sturdy chair, placing your feet flat on the floor, just slightly behind your knees. Lean slightly forward and keep your torso firm throughout this exercise.

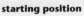

starting position

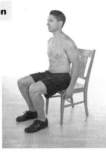

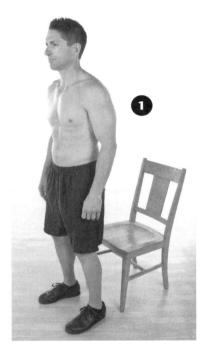

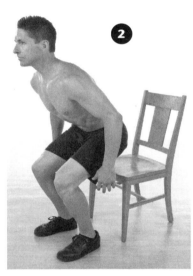

1 Slowly stand up without using your hands, if possible.

2 Lower yourself slowly into the chair.

Do not apply too much resistance with either of these steps.

STARTING POSITION: Sit toward the front of a chair with both feet flat on the floor.

starting position

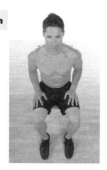

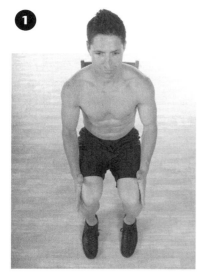

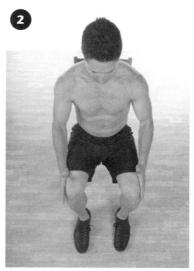

1 Place your hands on the outsides of your thighs near your knees.

2 Spread your legs a comfortable width as you resist the motion with your hands. Breathe comfortably.

3 Now place your hands on the insides of your thighs and resist the motion as you squeeze your legs together.

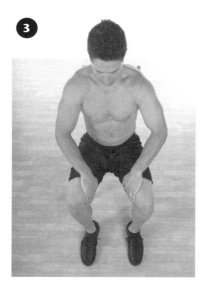

VARIATION: For the squeeze portion, you may place a foam roller between your thighs for extra resistance

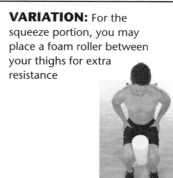

If you have long legs, roll up a towel and place it under your knees to raise them. If you find this exercise too difficult, try it without weights.

STARTING POSITION: Strap an ankle weight around each ankle and sit at the edge of a stable chair. Place your hands in a comfortable position. Inhale to begin.

starting position

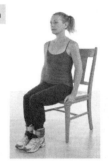

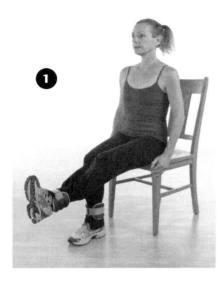

1 Exhale and slowly extend your left leg until it's straight, but not hyperextended. Hold for a count of 1–2.

2 Inhale and slowly return your leg to starting position.

Repeat, then switch sides.

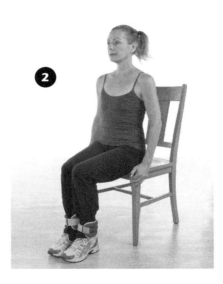

If you find this exercise too difficult, try it without weights.

STARTING POSITION: Strap an ankle weight around each ankle and sit in a chair with proper posture. Straighten your left leg by tightening the upper leg muscles. Inhale to begin.

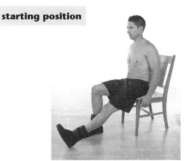

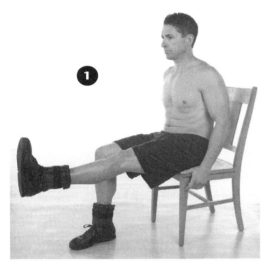

1 Keep your left leg straight as you exhale and lift it up so that it's parallel with the floor. Do not lean back as you lift your leg.

2 Inhale and slowly return the leg to the floor.

Repeat, then switch sides.

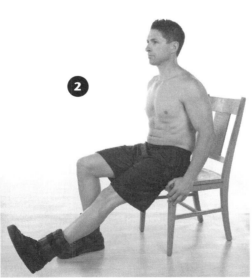

STARTING POSITION: Sit with proper posture in the middle of the chair. Wrap an exercise band around your right foot and hold an end of the band in each hand. Inhale to begin.

starting position

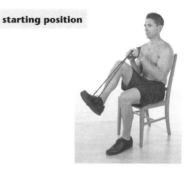

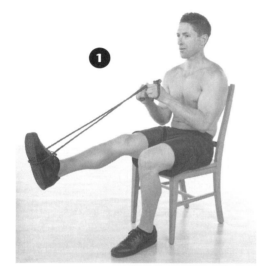

1 Exhale and slowly extend your right leg forward, but do not lock your knee.

2 Inhale and slowly return to starting position.

Repeat, then switch sides.

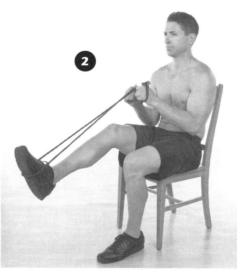

If you've had hip replacement surgery, this helps circulate the blood.

STARTING POSITION: Sit in a chair with proper posture. Extend your left leg and loop a band around your foot, crossing the band above your shin for safety. Keep your leg straight and your toes pointing straight up.

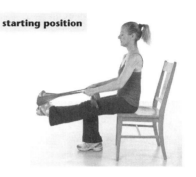

starting position

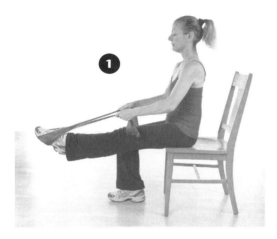

1 Point your foot away from you, against the band's resistance. Hold for a moment.

2 Return to starting position.

Repeat, then switch sides.

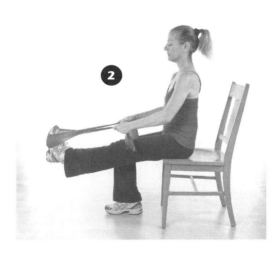

STARTING POSITION: Sit in a chair with proper posture.

starting position

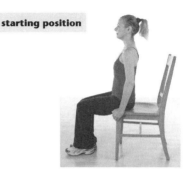

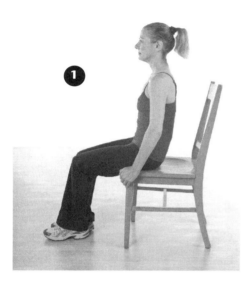

1 Slowly roll your tailbone under and hold the position for 3–5 seconds, concentrating on whether it increases or decreases pain. Remember where it feels the best.

2 Return to starting position, then slowly roll your tailbone backward, sticking your bottom back. Hold for 3–5 seconds.

Return to starting position. Repeat 5–10 times in each direction. However, proper execution is more important than reps here.

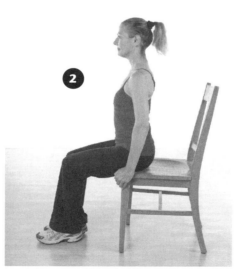

VARIATION: To make this exercise more challenging, perform the movement while sitting on a stability ball.

If you find this exercise too difficult, try it without weights.

STARTING POSITION: Strap an ankle weight around each ankle and lie on the right side of your body, positioning your body in a comfortable position so as to not hurt your back. You can bend your lower leg to reduce stress on your back. Rest your head on your right upper arm and straighten your top leg. Inhale to begin.

starting position

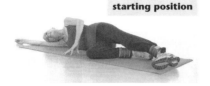

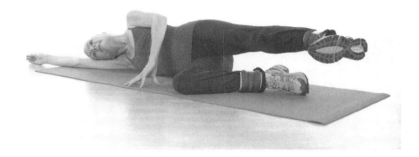

1 Keeping your left leg straight, exhale and lift it up to shoulder height.

2 Inhale and slowly return to starting position.

Repeat, then switch sides.

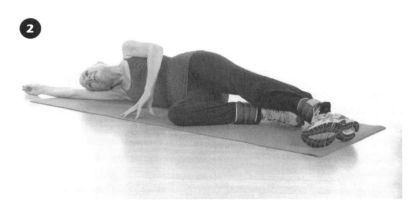

VARIATION: To perform this with an exercise band, tie the ends of the band together and loop it around both ankles.

floor series
reverse side-lying leg lift
inner thighs

If you find this exercise too difficult, try it without weights.

STARTING POSITION: Strap an ankle weight around each ankle and lie on the right side of your body. Rest your head on your right upper arm and straighten your lower leg. Bend your top leg and place the foot over and in front of your other leg; try to keep this foot flat on the floor. Place your other hand on the floor in front of your pelvis for support. Inhale to begin.

starting position

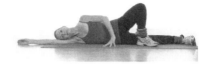

1

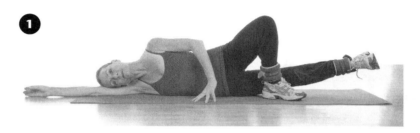

1 Keeping your lower leg straight, exhale and lift it as high as is comfortable and hold.

2 Inhale and lower to starting position.

Repeat, then switch sides.

2

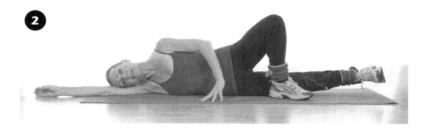

STARTING POSITION: Lie on your side with your bad leg on top and your toes pointing forward.

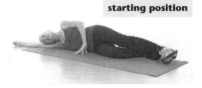

starting position

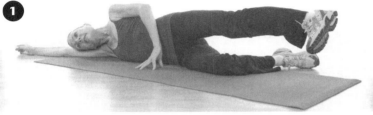

1

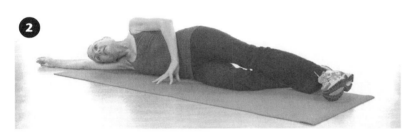

2

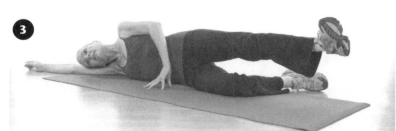

3

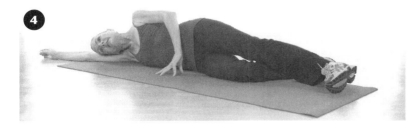

4

1 Point your toes down toward the floor. Hold for 1–3 seconds.

2 Return to starting position.

3 Point your toes up toward the ceiling. Hold for 1–3 seconds.

4 Return to starting position.

Repeat as tolerated, working up to 10 reps.

STARTING POSITION: Lie on your side with your body stacked: shoulder atop shoulder, hip atop hip, knee atop knee, ankle atop ankle.

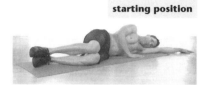

starting position

1

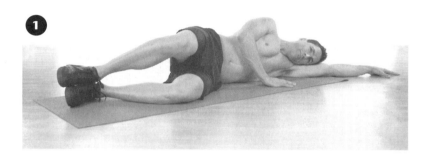

2

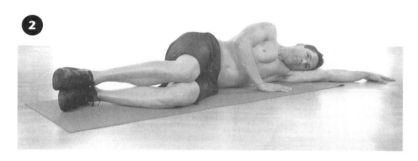

1 Gently open the top knee away from the bottom knee about 4–6 inches.

2 Return to starting position.

Repeat 3–10 times, as tolerated, then switch sides.

If you find this exercise too difficult, try it without weights.

CAUTION: Avoid this exercise if lying on your stomach is uncomfortable. However, placing a pillow or rolled-up towel under your hips does help most people.

STARTING POSITION: Strap an ankle weight around each ankle and lie face down on the floor. If necessary, position a pillow beneath your hips so that your back is in a comfortable neutral position. Rest your head on your forearms.

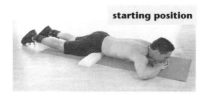

starting position

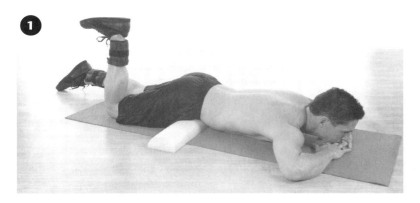

1 Slowly bring your right heel up toward your buttock, stopping when it reaches 90 degrees.

2 Slowly return your foot to starting position.

Repeat, then switch sides.

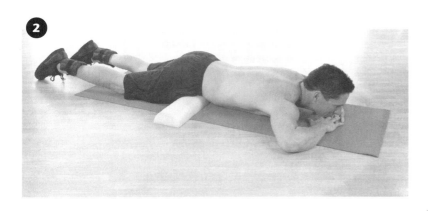

VARIATION: To perform this with an exercise band, tie the ends together and loop it around both ankles.

If you find this exercise too difficult, try it without weights.

STARTING POSITION: Strap an ankle weight around each ankle and get down on your hands and knees.

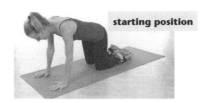

starting position

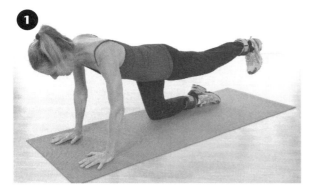

1 Keeping your back straight, extend your left leg straight back and lift it up parallel to the floor; make sure your upper leg is parallel to the floor throughout the exercise. Inhale to begin.

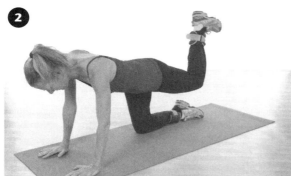

2 Exhale to bend your left knee and pull your heel toward your buttocks, stopping when you reach 90 degrees. Hold for a moment. If you feel a cramp coming on, stop and stretch your leg.

3 Inhale and extend your leg.

Repeat, then switch sides.

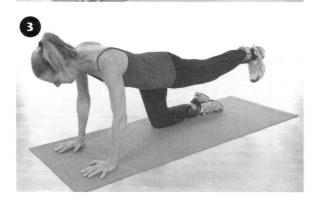

STARTING POSITION: Lie on your back with your feet flat on the floor and your arms alongside your body. Keep your core contracted and your lower back in neutral throughout the movement.

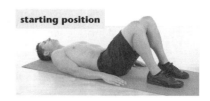

starting position

1

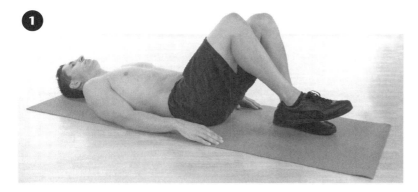

1 Imagining that a wire is pulling your knee upward, inhale and slowly lift your right foot an inch or two off the floor. The smaller the distance you lift the foot off the floor (such as leaving just enough space to slip a piece of paper under), the more challenging the move.

2

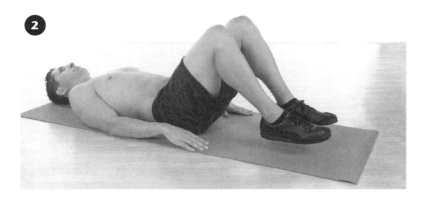

2 Exhale and slowly raise your left foot off the floor as you lower your right.

STARTING POSITION: Lie on your back with your feet flat on the floor and your arms alongside your body. Keeping your lower back neutral throughout the exercise, lift both legs off the floor as if resting them on an imaginary chair. Keep control of your core. Inhale to begin.

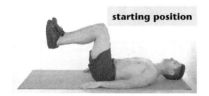

starting position

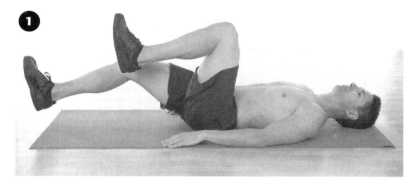

1 Without allowing your pelvis to rock or roll, exhale and contract your abdominal muscles as you press one leg forward and pull the other toward your chest.

2 Inhale and switch sides, pressing the other leg forward as you pull the forward leg back.

Continue alternating legs.

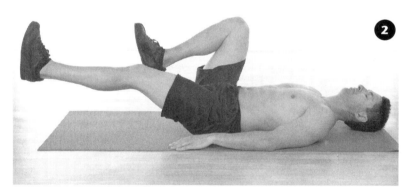

STARTING POSITION: Lie on your back with your feet flat on the floor and your arms crossed over your chest.

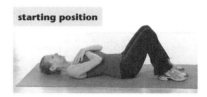

starting position

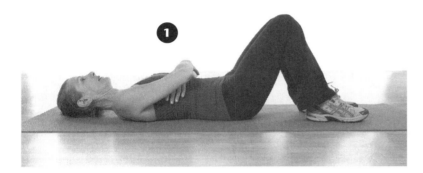

1 Press your lower back into the floor (the normal curve of your spine should be lying flat so not even a piece of paper can slide between your back and the floor). Hold for a count of 1–2–3 and then relax.

floor series
pelvic lift

STARTING POSITION: Lie on your back with your feet flat on the floor and your arms along your sides. Press the small of your back into the floor as you tighten your core muscles. Find your neutral spine position and maintain this position throughout the exercise. Inhale to begin.

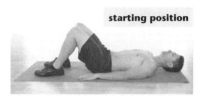

starting position

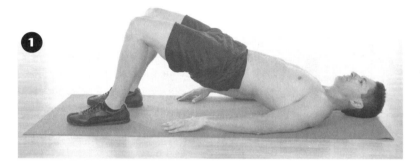

1 Exhale and lift your hips and lower back off the floor. Hold this position for a moment, keeping your pelvic area stationary.

2 Inhale and lower yourself to the floor.

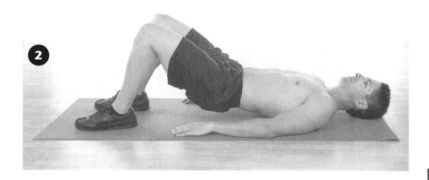

VARIATION: Perform the exercise after you've placed a band over your pelvis and secured the band in each hand at a position for ideal resistance.

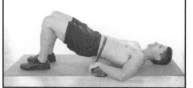

This advanced exercise will improve core stabilization of the whole midsection area. Make sure you can do the regular Pelvic Lift (page 102) before attempting this.

CAUTION: If you feel a cramp coming on, stop and stretch your hamstrings.

starting position

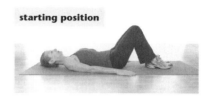

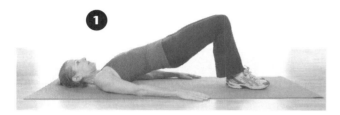

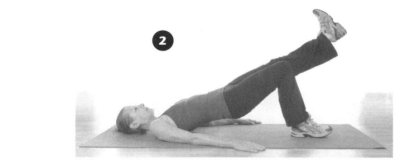

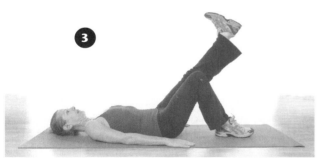

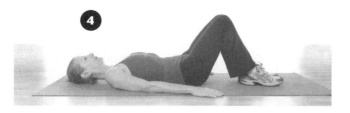

STARTING POSITION: Lie on your back with your knees bent, feet flat on the floor and arms alongside your body. Inhale to begin.

1 Exhale and press your feet into the ground to slowly lift your rear end and lower back off the floor; you will ultimately form a straight line from your shoulders to your hips.

2 Slowly straighten your left leg from the knee joint until it's diagonal to the ground; hold this position for 5–10 seconds.

3 Inhale and slowly lower your hips to the ground.

4 Place your left foot on the ground.

Repeat the sequence using the other leg.

This advanced exercise must be done properly to engage all the muscles of the core.

CAUTION: Do not perform this move if you have high blood pressure or a hernia.

POSITION: Assume a modified push-up position by placing your forearms shoulder-width apart on the floor and extending your legs behind you to balance on the balls of your feet. Contract your midsection to prevent from sagging. Maintain this position for the recommended time, breathing comfortably; do not hold your breath.

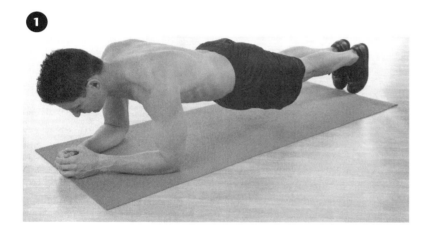

VARIATION: For an extra challenge, try lifting one leg and then the other.

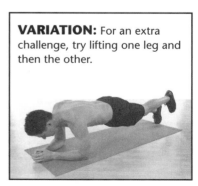

This advanced exercise requires total mind-body engagement of the core.

CAUTION: Do not perform this if you have shoulder joint issues or cardiovascular concerns.

POSITION: Lying on the left side of your body, position your elbow under your shoulder to prop yourself up. Inhale to begin.

starting position

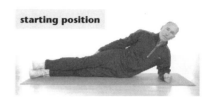

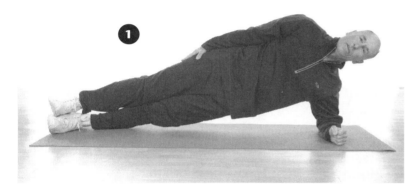

1 Exhale and contract your midsection, pressing your forearm into the floor to lift your hips off the floor. Assume a straight line from your ankles to your shoulders. Maintain this position for the recommended time. Come down to rest, then switch sides.

STARTING POSITION: Lie with your upper back on a stability ball and your bottom and your feet flat on the floor. Inhale to begin.

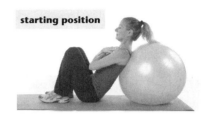

starting position

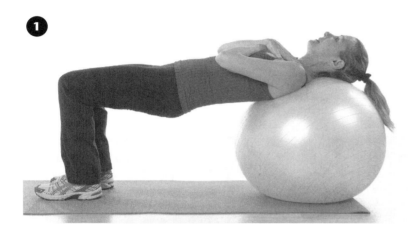

1 Exhale as you slowly lift your bottom up to a neutral height or parallel with the floor. Squeeze your gluteal muscles and be careful of hamstring cramps.

Inhale and slowly lower your bottom and repeat.

STARTING POSITION: Lie on your back with your heels resting on a ball and your arms along your sides. Press the small of your back into the floor as you tighten your core muscles. Find your neutral spine position and maintain this position throughout the exercise. Inhale to begin.

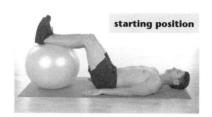

starting position

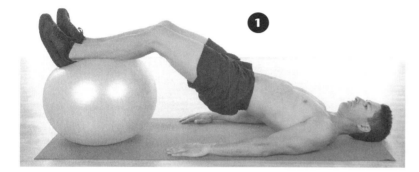

1

1 Exhale and lift your hips and lower back off the floor. Hold this position for a moment, keeping your pelvic area stationary.

2 Inhale and lower yourself to the floor.

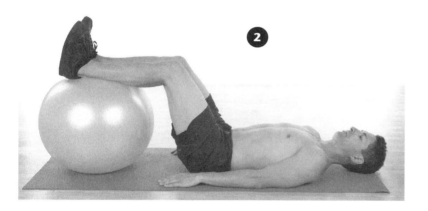

2

STARTING POSITION: Lie with your upper back on a stability ball and your feet on the floor, creating a table-top position parallel to the floor. Maintain neutral spine position throughout the movement by tightening your abs. Inhale to begin.

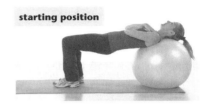

starting position

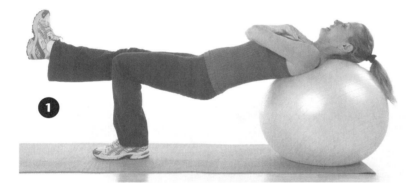

1 Exhale and extend your right leg straight out in front of you, as high as you can without wobbling.

2 Inhale and return to starting position.

Alternate legs.

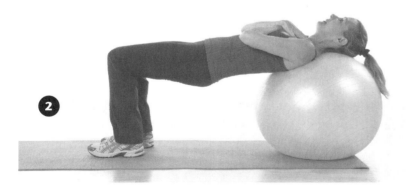

This advanced motion teaches you to better control your core when doing compound motions.

STARTING POSITION: Lie on your back in proper neutral spine posture and place your heels on the ball. Your arms can be extended along your sides for support. Inhale to begin.

starting position

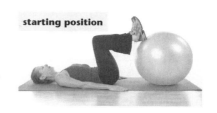

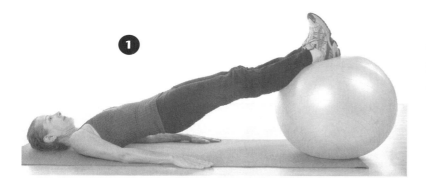

1 Maintaining neutral spine, exhale and extend your legs to roll the ball outward, stopping before you lose neutral spine; hold.

2 Inhale and slowly roll the ball back to starting position.

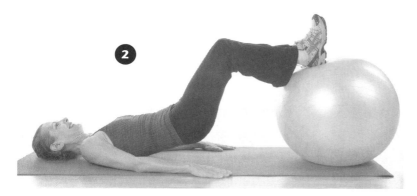

MODIFICATION: You can do this using one leg at a time until you're able to use both legs.

STARTING POSITION: Lie face down with your upper body on the ball and your legs extended behind you, toes on the floor. Place your hands on the floor. Inhale to begin.

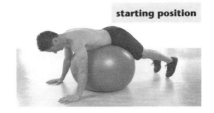

starting position

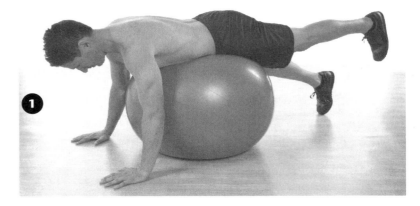

1 Exhale and slowly lift one leg behind you and hold for 5 seconds.

2 Inhale and return to starting position.

Switch sides and repeat.

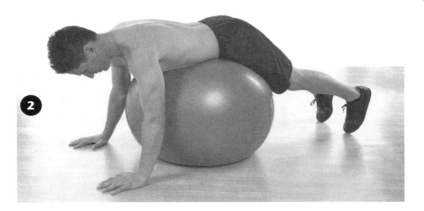

VARIATION: For an extra challenge, try the exercise with one or both arms off the floor.

Make sure you have plenty of space to perform this move.

STARTING POSITION: Lie face down with your belly button centered over the middle of the ball. Place your hands on the floor for support; keep your legs extended behind you and toes on the floor. Maintain neutral spine position throughout the movement by tightening your abs. Inhale to begin.

starting position

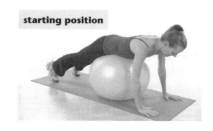

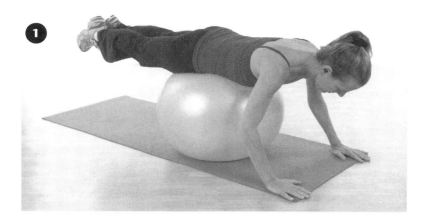

1 Exhale and lift both legs up to the height of your rear end and hold for 3–5 seconds.

Inhale and slowly lower to starting position and reposition your body, checking for neutral spine position before repeating.

VARIATION: This can also be done by lifting one leg at a time.

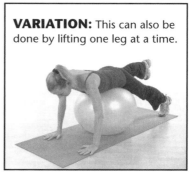

STARTING POSITION: Lie face down and comfortably balanced on a stability ball. Place your hands on the floor; keep your legs extended behind you and toes on the floor. Maintain neutral spine position throughout the movement by tightening your abs. Inhale to begin.

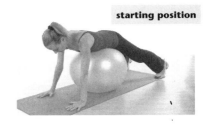
starting position

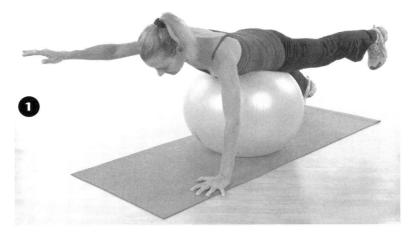

1 Exhale and slowly lift your right arm and left leg as high as is tolerated, but no higher than your shoulders.

2 Inhale and return to starting position.

Switch sides, slowly lifting your left arm and right leg. The goal is 5–15 reps while maintaining proper form.

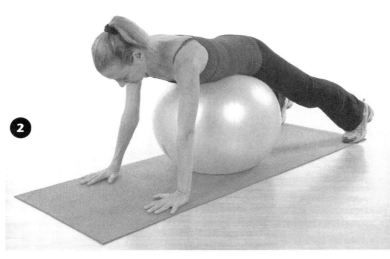

VARIATION: For an extra challenge, try this with both arms raised.

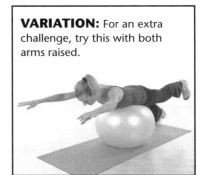

Be sure to find a safe, spacious place to perform this move.

STARTING POSITION: Lie face down with your belly button centered over the middle of the ball. Place your hands and toes lightly on the floor for support. Maintain neutral spine position throughout the movement by tightening your abs. Inhale to begin.

starting position

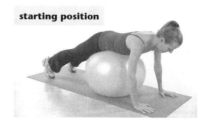

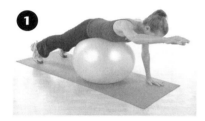

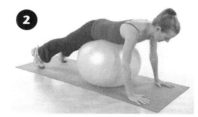

1 Exhale and slowly lift your right arm to shoulder height and hold for 1–3 seconds.

2 Inhale and slowly lower to starting position.

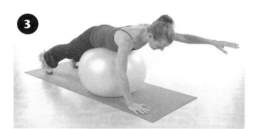

3 Exhale and slowly lift your left arm to shoulder height and hold for 1–3 seconds.

4 Inhale and slowly lower to starting position.

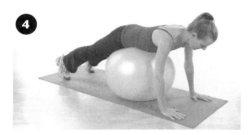

5 Exhale and lift both arms and hold for 1–3 seconds.

Repeat the sequence 5 times if possible.

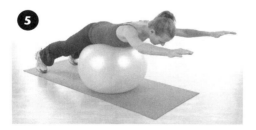

This advanced exercise fosters proper upper back posture and reverses the rounded/hunched back that comes with overly inflexible chest muscles. It also requires core strength and balance.

STARTING POSITION: Lie face down with your belly button centered over the middle of the ball; raise your legs until they're parallel to the floor. Your fingertips provide only light assistance for balance. Inhale to begin.

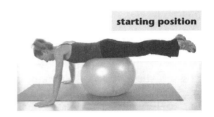

starting position

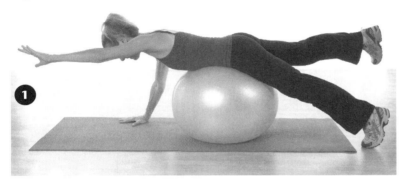

1 Exhale and lift your left arm parallel to the ground and touch your left toes to the ground; hold.

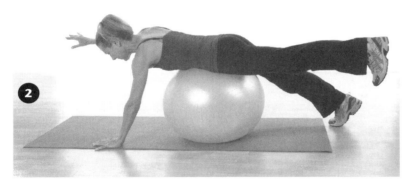

2 Now switch so that your other arm comes up and your other foot goes down.

Continue switching, maintaining proper form.

STARTING POSITION: Stand with your feet shoulder-width apart and about 12 to 18 inches from a wall so that you can place a stability ball against your back.

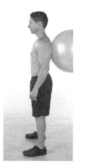

starting position

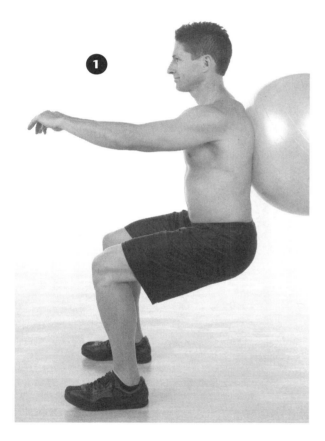

1 Exhale as you squat down as far as is comfortable, with your knees pointing straight ahead. Your knees should not go farther than 90 degrees.

Return to starting position. Repeat 2–10 times.

STARTING POSITION: Sit on a stability ball and maintain proper posture. Imagine that the ball is the face of a clock.

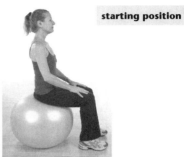

starting position

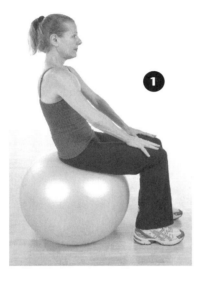

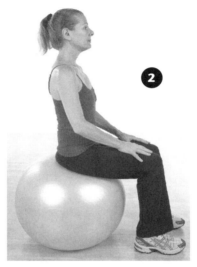

1 Slowly tuck your tailbone under, attempting to move your tailbone to 12 o'clock. Hold for 1–3 seconds.

2 Return to neutral position.

3 Slowly roll your tailbone backward toward 6 o'clock, sticking your bottom back.

4 Return to neutral position.

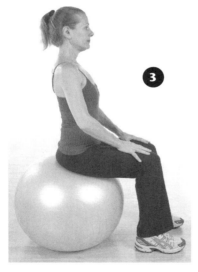

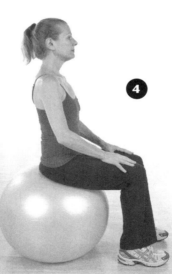

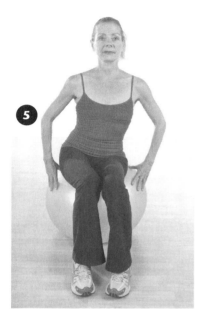

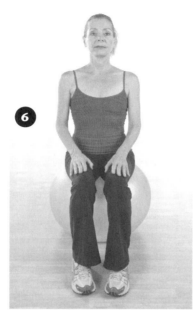

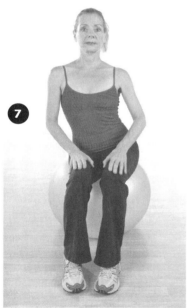

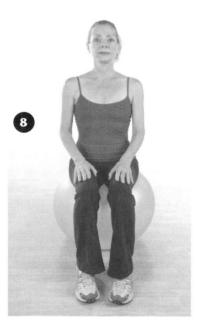

5 Slowly roll your right hip to the right (toward 3 o'clock).

6 Return to neutral position.

7 Slowly roll your left hip to the left (toward 9 o'clock).

8 Return to neutral position.

Roll as far as is tolerated in each direction and increase the range of motion as you improve. Only repeat the series if you can do it perfectly.

STARTING POSITION: Lie on your back with your heels resting on the ball and your arms alongside your body. Keep your lower back neutral throughout the exercise. Inhale to begin.

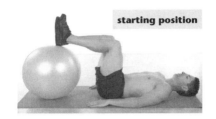

starting position

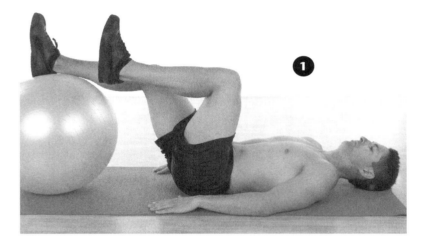

1

1 Without allowing your pelvis to rock or roll, exhale and contract your abdominal muscles as you press one leg forward and pull the other toward your chest.

2 Inhale and switch sides, pressing the other leg forward as you pull the forward leg back.

Continue alternating legs.

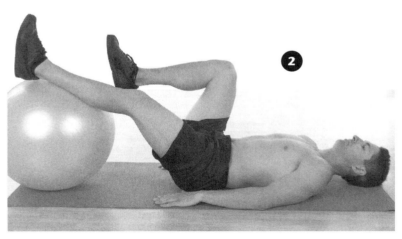

2

This exercise will enhance dynamic balance and power.

STARTING POSITION: Stand with your feet about shoulder-width apart in a solid athletic stance.

starting position

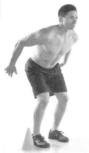

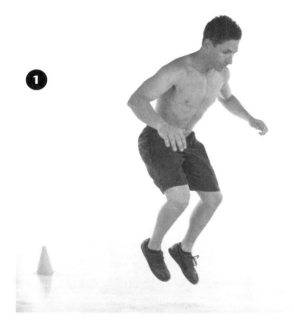

1–2 Jump forward, landing on both feet; absorb the shock and maintain balance by keeping your knees soft. Hold for a moment.

Jump backwards.

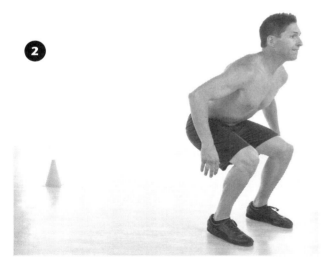

sports-ready series
lateral jump & hold
legs

120

This movement is designed for athletes who play sports that require a lot of lateral movement, such as tennis. Be mindful of any increase in discomfort; do not perform until fully recovered and do not perform more than two times per week.

STARTING POSITION: Stand with your feet about shoulder-width apart in a solid athletic stance.

starting position

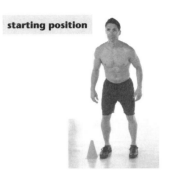

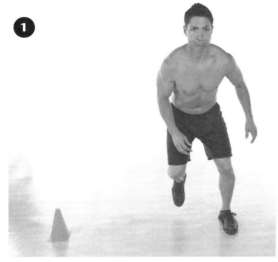

1 Jump sideways to the left, landing on your left foot and maintaining your balance. Hold for a moment.

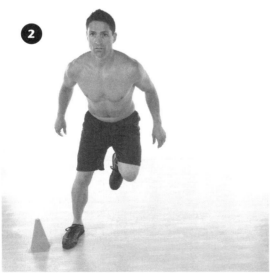

2 Jump to the right, landing on your right foot and maintaining your balance. Hold for a moment.

Continue jumping left and right, holding for a moment before performing the next jump.

This exercise will enhance dynamic balance and power. You'll need enough space to move forward. Be mindful of any increase in discomfort; do not perform until fully recovered and do not perform more than two times per week.

STARTING POSITION: Stand on your right foot.

starting position

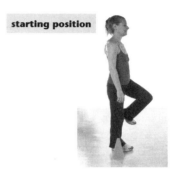

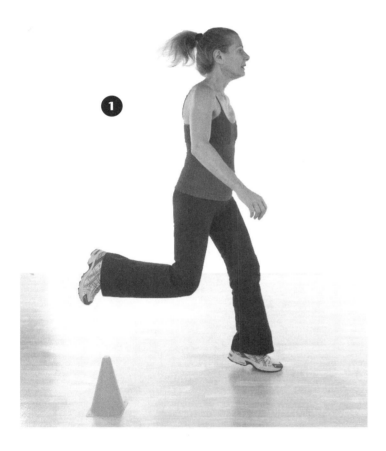

1 Hop forward, landing on your left foot; absorb the shock and maintain balance by keeping your knee soft. Hold for a moment.

Continue hopping forward, this time landing on your right foot. Repeat, alternating feet.

VARIATION: If space is an issue, hop back to your starting position and then hop forward with your other foot.

The name of this exercise is misleading because it does not actually feel like "play." This advanced activity challenges the aerobic and anaerobic systems of the body and should not be performed until you have an excellent baseline of fitness and health. This exercise also helps improve performance times. You'll need to go to a local track to do this.

Be mindful of any increase in discomfort; do not perform until fully recovered and do not perform more than two times per week.

STARTING POSITION: Select a starting line at the point where the track straightens out. Have a stopwatch available to measure times if desired.

1 Sprint as fast as you can down the straightaways.

2 As you enter the curve, slow down the pace dramatically by either jogging or walking the curve.

3 When you're ready, sprint the straightaway as fast as you want.

4 Recover around the curve.

TIPS: This workout should only be done once or twice a week, well separated by recovery time to avoid injury. This same concept can be applied to biking or swimming (i.e., sprint a set distance and then slow down).

This exercise helps your footwork become more fluid. Be mindful of any increase in discomfort; do not perform until fully recovered and do not perform more than two times per week.

STARTING POSITION: Place two targets a good distance from each other. Start at one end, keeping your feet wide and center of gravity low.

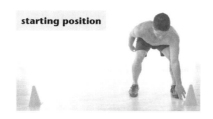

starting position

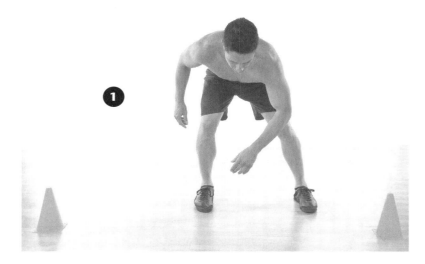

1 Keeping your weight low, shuffle smoothly to the other target.

2 Touch the target before shuffling back to the other side.

Continue shuffling for the recommended amount of time.

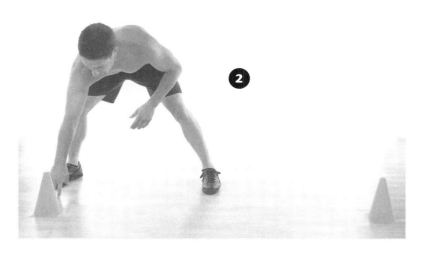

This activity improves lateral jumping power. The series of targets can be created by drawing circles on the ground with chalk or placing down pieces of tape or other markers. Be mindful of any increase in discomfort; do not perform until fully recovered and do not perform more than two times per week.

CAUTION: Avoid this activity if you have any orthopedic issues.

STARTING POSITION: Stand inside the circle or on a target.

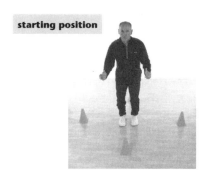

starting position

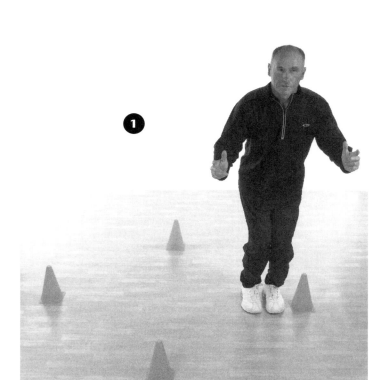

1 Jump to the next target and hold.

After you've jumped the series of targets, jump in the other direction.

Repeat quickly to develop power and agility.

VARIATION: You can have a partner call out different targets to land on in an unpredictable manner. This can also be performed on one leg.

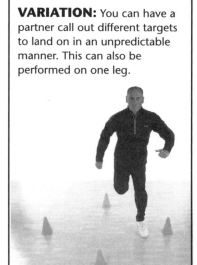

CAUTION: *If you have knee or balance issues, do not perform this exercise. Be mindful of any increase in discomfort; do not perform until fully recovered and do not perform more than two times per week.*

STARTING POSITION: With your feet on either side of a marker, stand tall with a solid athletic stance.

starting position

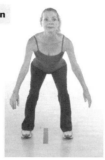

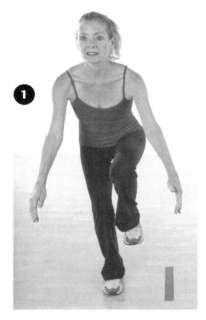

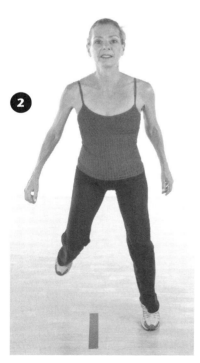

1 Raise your left heel to your rear end and hop to the right.

2 Return to starting position for a second to regain balance, then quickly raise your right heel to your rear end and hop to the left.

Repeat as quickly as possible for the recommended time or until fatigued.

VARIATION: If you're more advanced, do not stand on both legs—just quickly shift from left to right legs. For the super-advanced, place a 2x4 on the floor and hop left and right over it.

sports-ready series
double-leg jump

Be mindful of any increase in discomfort; do not perform until fully recovered and do not perform more than two times per week.

CAUTION: If you have weak ankles, knees or poor balance, start this exercise in the pool.

STARTING POSITION: Stand in an athletic stance.

starting position

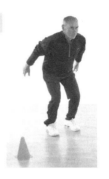

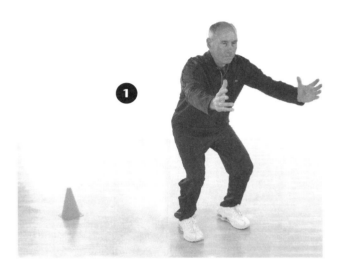

1 Jump as far forward as is comfortable, landing on both feet while maintaining your balance. Make sure you push evenly off of both legs.

2 Jump backwards to the starting point, landing on both legs.

Repeat quickly to develop power and agility.

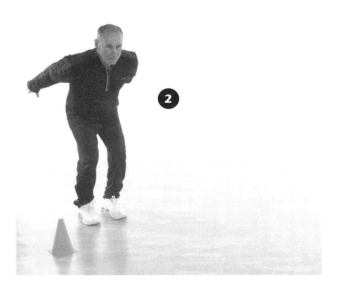

Be mindful of any increase in discomfort; do not perform until fully recovered and do not perform more than two times per week.

CAUTION: If you have weak ankles, knees or poor balance, start this exercise in the pool.

STARTING POSITION: Stand on your left leg.

starting position

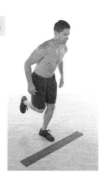

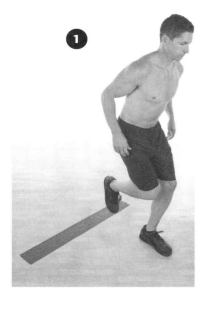

1 Jump as far forward as is comfortable, landing on your left foot while maintaining your balance.

2 Jump backwards to the starting point, landing on your left foot.

Switch sides. Repeat quickly to develop power and agility.

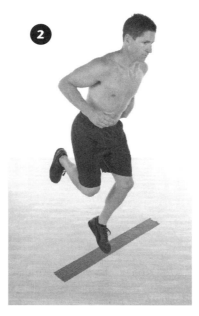

MODIFICATION: As you advance, try to jump for height instead of distance.

index

other ulysses press books

Healthy Shoulder Handbook: 100 Exercises for Treating & Preventing Frozen Shoulder, Rotator Cuff & Other Common Injuries
Dr. Karl Knopf, $14.95

With easy-to-do stretches and carefully designed weight-training programs, this book includes everything needed to turn a troublesome shoulder into a sturdy and strong joint.

Stretching for 50+: A Customized Program for Increasing Flexibility, Avoiding Injury & Enjoying an Active Lifestyle
Dr. Karl Knopf, $13.95

Shows how to maintain and improve flexibility by incorporating additional stretching into one's life. Covering all the muscle groups, this book offers special programs catering to every fitness level.

Total Sports Conditioning for Athletes 50+: Workouts for Staying at the Top of Your Game
Dr. Karl Knopf, $14.95

Getting older doesn't mean losing to younger competitors! *Total Sports Conditioning for Athletes 50+* provides sport-specific workouts that allow aging athletes to maintain the flexibility, strength, and speed needed to win.

Weights for 50+: Building Strength, Staying Healthy & Enjoying an Active Lifestyle
Dr. Karl Knopf, $14.95

Shows how easy it is for anyone—at any age—to lift weights, stay fit and active, and also guard against osteoporosis, diabetes and heart disease.

The Anatomy of Martial Arts: An Illustrated Guide to the Muscles Used for Each Strike, Kick & Throw
Norman G. Link & Lily Chou, $16.95

The perfect training supplement for martial artists, this book's detailed anatomical drawings show exactly what is happening inside the body while it's performing a physical movement.

Complete Krav Maga: The Ultimate Guide to Over 230 Self-Defense and Combative Techniques
Darren Levine & John Whitman, $21.95

Krav Maga is an easy-to-learn yet highly effective art of self-defense. *Complete Krav Maga* details every aspect of the system, including hand-to-hand combat moves and weapons defense techniques.

Ellie Herman's Pilates Workbook on the Ball: Illustrated Step-by-Step Guide
Ellie Herman, $14.95

Combines the powerful slimming and shaping effects of Pilates with the low-impact, high-intensity workout of the ball.

Functional Training for Athletes at All Levels: Workouts for Agility, Speed & Power
James C. Radcliffe, $15.95

Teaches all athletes the functional training exercises that will produce the best results in their sport by mimicking the actual movements they utilize in that sport. With these unique programs, athletes can simultaneously improve posture, balance, stability and mobility.

Get On It!: BOSU® Balance Trainer Workouts for Core Strength & a Super Toned Body

Colleen Craig, Miriane Taylor & Jane Aronovitch, $14.95

Shows how to tap the power of the BOSU® to reshape one's whole body while strengthening the core and stabilizing muscles.

Plyometrics for Athletes at All Levels: A Training Guide for Explosive Speed & Power

Neal Pire, $15.95

Provides an easy-to-understand explanation of why plyometrics works, the sports-training research behind it, and how to integrate plyometrics into an overall fitness program.

Total Heart Rate Training: Customize & Maximize Your Workout Using a Heart Rate Monitor

Joe Friel, $15.95

Shows anyone participating in aerobic sports, from novice to expert, how to increase the effectiveness of his or her workout by utilizing a heart rate monitor.

Ultimate Conditioning for Tennis: 130 Exercises for Power, Agility & Quickness

Alan Pearson, $15.95

Offers exercises for building a rock-solid physical foundation from which a player can develop a winning game. The clearly illustrated drills will help players at all levels improve their game.

To order these books call 800-377-2542 or 510-601-8301, fax 510-601-8307, e-mail ulysses@ulyssespress.com, or write to Ulysses Press, P.O. Box 3440, Berkeley, CA 94703. All retail orders are shipped free of charge. California residents must include sales tax. Allow two to three weeks for delivery.

acknowlegdments

It is a joy to work with such a team of professionals, without whose skill and expertise this book would not have been possible. I would like to sincerely thank Lily Chou and Claire Chun, whose attention to detail and ability to explain complex concepts in user-friendly terms is without parallel. Thanks also to models Brian Goodell and Toni Silver for their patience, and to Austin Forbord and his team at Rapt Productions, who were able to capture the essence of the exercises so well. I'd like to thank acquisitions editor Keith Riegert for his vision. Lastly, a special note of appreciation to my son Chris Knopf, who served as my fact checker. Special thanks to my wife Margaret of 30-plus years for so graciously allowing me private time in the living room to write this and other books.